Postmemory, Psychoanalysis and Holocaust Ghosts

Through the collection of letters sent by members of a Jewish family between 1923 and 1942, this fascinating book explores phenomenological and
psychoanalytical aspects of the Holocaust and its associated trauma, and
the impact on future generations of the same family.

This book charts a postmemorial study of the Cohen family of Salonica
which branched out to Paris and Tel-Aviv during the 1920s and 1930s. The
exploration of the contents of four boxes containing hundreds of letters,
pictures and other documents portray a microhistory of one family that was
once a part of a thriving community. Showing how the shadows of trauma
can be passed through the generations, the book uncovers the tragedies that
befell the Cohen family, and how the discovery of these materials has affected existing family members.

In an intriguing work of postmemory research and analysis, this book
appeals to both scholars of the holocaust and psychoanalysts interested in
the unconscious impact of history.

Rony Alfandary, PhD, is a clinical social worker, photographer and lec-
turer at the University of Haifa and Bar-Ilan University in Israel. He is the
Director of the Programme of Psychoanalytic Psychotherapy at Bar-Ilan
University. He has published prose and poetry as well as several works of
non-fiction including *Exile and Return: A Psychoanalytic Study of Lawrence
Durrell's The Alexandria Quartet* (Routledge).

Postmemory, Psychoanalysis and Holocaust Ghosts

The Salonica Cohen Family and Trauma Across Generations

Rony Alfandary

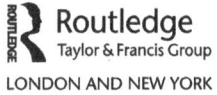

Routledge
Taylor & Francis Group

LONDON AND NEW YORK

First published 2022
by Routledge
2 Park Square, Milton Park, Abingdon, Oxon OX14 4RN

and by Routledge
605 Third Avenue, New York, NY 10158

Routledge is an imprint of the Taylor & Francis Group, an informa business

British Library Cataloguing-in-Publication Data
A catalogue record for this book is available from the British Library

Library of Congress Cataloging-in-Publication Data
Names: Alfandary, Rony, author.
Title: Postmemory, psychoanalysis and Holocaust ghosts : the Salonica Cohen family and trauma across generations / Rony Alfandary.
Description: Milton Park, Abingdon, Oxon ; New York, NY : Routledge, [2021] | Includes bibliographical references and index. |
Identifiers: LCCN 2021003396 (print) | LCCN 2021003397 (ebook) | ISBN 9780367491994 (hardback) | ISBN 9780367491741 (paperback) | ISBN 9781003189121 (ebook)
Subjects: LCSH: Holocaust survivors—Greece—Thessalonikē. | Holocaust, Jewish (1939–1945)—Psychological aspects. | Holocaust survivors—Family relationships. | Cohen family. | Holocaust, Jewish (1939–1945)—Greece—Thessalonikē. | World War, 1939–1945—Atrocities—Greece—Thessalonikē. | Holocaust, Jewish (1939–1945)—Influence. | Thessalonikē (Greece)—Ethnic relations.
Classification: LCC RC451.4.H62 A43 2021 (print) | LCC RC451.4.H62 (ebook) | DDC 940.53/180922—dc23
LC record available at https://lccn.loc.gov/2021003396
LC ebook record available at https://lccn.loc.gov/2021003397

ISBN: 978-0-367-49199-4 (hbk)
ISBN: 978-0-367-49174-1 (pbk)
ISBN: 978-1-003-18912-1 (ebk)

Typeset in Times New Roman
by codeMantra

Souvenir de mis ermanos deportados a la Segunda Guerra al 1942. Quero yo, vouestra madre, y nona Parente, que vos acodrech siempre de eyos, que la familia Cohen non suembare a vouestro aouvenir. Vouestra madre y nona.

Rita Cohen Parenti[1]

Note

1 This is the inscription Rita Parenti left inside the photo album she had kept of her brothers and sister and their families who were murdered in Auschwitz. It is written in Ladino (a rich and proverbial Judaeo-Spanish dialect used as the main written and spoken language of Jewish communities in the Balkan and other countries where Jews were expelled from Spain in the fifteenth century. The core vocabulary of Judaeo-Spanish is Old Spanish, and it has numerous elements from Ottoman Turkish and Semitic vocabulary such as Hebrew, Aramaic and Arabic): "A souvenir from my siblings who were deported during WW2 in 1942. I am your mother and grandmother and I want you to remember me and the Cohen family always, so they are not lost from your memory. Your mother and Grandmother".

Contents

Figures

Acknowledgements

When I set out to write this book, my mother's complaint that she had never seen a photograph of her maternal grandfather, Shabtai Cohen, who died years before she was born, kept echoing in my mind. The work on this book has at least done that – through my research, I was able to identify two photographs of him. She now knows what he looked like....

This book is first dedicated to my mother, whose burden concerning the loss is unremitting. A very special thanks goes to my sister, whose support has been invaluable, and to my father, a refugee himself, who quietly observed and approved of my efforts. It is also dedicated to my uncles, aunts and cousins, all part of the Cohen–Parenti tribe. I hope it will serve us all in preserving the memory of the family we had lost. I also hope that it will help us all to become better human beings. Especially I want to thank my aunt, Eli Parran, who went over the MS in its early stages and made invaluable suggestions. Eli's late husband, my dear uncle Benjamin, produced a booklet of some of the letters twenty years ago that was the foundation upon which this book is based. A special thanks to my French aunt, Mireille Florent, without whom most of the letters would not have been found and to her daughter, my cousin Marianne Leloir, who translated some of the letters as well as being a soulmate along the path. Many thanks to my dear friend Dr. Emanuel Cohen, who helped with the translations of many of the letters.

Many people inspired me along the way in this project. My good friend Richard Pine of the Durrell Library of Corfu offered his generosity, gentleness and superb mastery of the language in bringing the final MS to its publishable state. The good people at Routledge who saved no effort in bringing this project to its final stage. My friends and colleagues, Prof. Laura Hobson Faure (without whose initial advice at a time of turmoil, this book may have not been written at all), Prof. Judy Tydor Baumel-Schwartz (my partner in other postmemory projects), Prof. Shmuel Rafael (who first gave a stage to a lecture concerning this topic at Bar-Ilan University), my buddy Yakir Elkariv (with whom I have been having imaginative and original conversations about writing and other things since 1978) and my dear friend Dr. Dominic Green (whose beautiful foreword honours this book). Many other friends, relatives and colleagues offered support and I apologize for not being able to name them all one by one. Thank you all.

The thoughts about my great uncles and aunt, their spouses and children, to whom this book is dedicated, who were murdered by the Nazis and their accomplices, accompanied me along the way. I hope this book does some justice to their memory, as well as to the memory of all the victims of the Nazi regime. I hope that I have made true my vow to my beloved grandmother, Rita, *we will never forget them*.

Finally, and mostly, my wife Didi and our sons, Dori and Eyal, who saw me struggle with the task and helped me with their constant warmth, love and support. You make this world a better place.

October 2020

Foreword

Dominic Green

A historian is someone who reads other people's letters. There are names for this sort of behaviour, most of them pejorative, but if the letters belong to the dead, then it is permitted and even praised. Yet, it isn't always harmless. Anyone who has assembled a family history recalls the pained expressions from the elderly relative squirming under interrogation, the evasions and changes of subject over the teacups and fruitcake, the implicit request not to bring the dead back to life.

Historians dream of having Rony Alfandary's luck: a series of boxes containing photographs, postcards and letters fall one by one into his lap from some dusty corner of a house in Provence. But to have Alfandary's luck, you must first have his misfortune: to be the heir of unspeakable sorrow. The Germans and their local collaborators murdered his grandmother Rita's family, the Cohens of Salonica in Greece. Rita Cohen survived because she and her husband had emigrated to the Land of Israel before the war. Another survivor, the sister-in-law of Rita's brother Leon, kept those boxes of material, but seemed unable to destroy or release them. Nothing is free when the psychological investigation is shadowed by lives foreshortened, when the human evidence has been hunted down and destroyed and when the archival tracings that each of us leaves in our wake turn out to have been written on water.

"The past is never dead. It's not even past", William Faulkner observed in *Requiem for a Nun*. Faulkner set that novel in 1938: the year of Munich; the year that Rita's mother, the matriarch Rachelle Bourla Cohen, died in Salonica; the year that Stefan Zweig, the peerless evoker of the "world of yesterday", suggested that the historian, aspiring to create a narrative from the fragmentary and arbitrary survivals of the physical record, must resort to the "free art of psychological investigation".

How do you reconstruct a story whose materials are smashed to fragments? Carlo Ginzburg famously compared the detective methodologies of Sigmund Freud, Sherlock Holmes and the art historian Giovanno Morelli. One of the peculiarities of the historian's craft, and the peculiar rewards of reading a book like this one, is the pleasures of the detective story: puzzling out the relationships between the shards of information, discovering the motivations of the characters and exposing the enormity of the crime. I won't discuss the details of Rony Alfandary's story here: much of the pleasure, and much of the horror too, lies in reading it for yourself. But I will note that he has accomplished something miraculous: he has turned names into characters and characters into stories. He has, as Isaiah's injunction and the name of Israel's Shoah archive say, supplied *yad v'shem*: "a sign and a name" to the unnamed and unburied dead.

*

No historical method gives greater weight to the weight of the past than the Austro-German fusion of the methods of Otto von Ranke and Sigmund Freud. Ranke believed that meticulous narrative reconstruction of the archives could show us the past *wie es eigentlich gewessen*: "as it really was". Freud, no less optimistic in his way, believed in the meticulous narrative reconstruction of the inner life. Both created templates for what are now called *microhistories*, highly detailed reconstructions whose resonances elucidate the wider history of their age.

The derailing of modern history by other Austro-Germans meant that psychohistory, as it became known, was developed in the universities of the United States, not Germany or Austria, just as the subsequent development of psychoanalysis occurred in Hampstead and the Upper West Side. For fifteen years, I lived within walking distance of the Freud Museum in Hampstead. I read books by Freud, I read books about Freud, I took pride in living in the street where Anna Freud had lived, I knew where Melanie Klein had lived, I laughed knowingly at the oral implications when I walked past the statue of Freud outside the Tavistock Clinic and saw that the cigarette butt that some well-informed comedian had inserted into his lips was still there and I read scholarly articles on the restoration of Freud's couch – but I never visited his house-museum.

Freud, who delayed visiting Rome, would have understood. When I was living within walking distance of the Freud Museum, a transplant symbolic of the wide history of his age, I was living in the same streets that my maternal grandparents had grown up in. One day, reading Stephen Spender's account of serving as a fireman during the Blitz, I realized that the explosions and fires Spender was describing were the ones that had destroyed the building in whose replacement I now live. I was experiencing the difference between psychological reality and historical narrative that Freud had described in *Civilization and its Discontents*.

Freud proposes the "fantastic supposition" that Rome was "not a human dwelling-place, but a mental entity with just as long and varied a past history". Nothing is erased, and each stage of its development co-exists in the same geography. Not only would the palaces of the Caesars be still standing on the Palatine, or "beautiful statues were still standing in the colonnade of the Castle of St. Angelo, as they were up to its siege by the Goths". It would also imply the physically impossible but psychically common. Where the Palazzo Caffarelli stands, there would also be the Temple of Jupiter Capitolinus, "not merely in its latest form, moreover, as the Romans of the Caesars saw it, but also in its earliest shape, when it still wore an Etruscan design and was adorned with terra-cotta antifixae". When we see the Coliseum, we would at the same time see the Golden House. We would see the current Pantheon, built by Hadrian, but also the original edifice of Agrippa. In an overlay familiar from religious history, the "same ground would support the church of Santa Maria sopra Minerva and the old temple over which it was built".

Historians have a boundless appetite for the past, but that can be too much of a bad thing. This is the plight that history placed Rony Alfandary as a young man. Like the mental overlay of the Palazzo Caffarelli and the Temple of Jupiter in Freud's mind, it is not possible to separate what was personal to Alfandary – his grandmother's need for her murdered family to remain "awake" in memory – from the "human dwelling-place" of collective memory, written history and formal remembrance. "History, Stephen said, is a nightmare from which I am trying to awake", Joyce wrote in *A Portrait of the Artist as Young Man*.

Freud opened *The Interpretation of Dreams* with a line from the *Aeneid*, spoken by Juno in her unbearable distress: "If I cannot move the gods, I will summon the underworld". It is impossible to bring the dead back to life by some "fantastic supposition", to vivify the names of the Cohen siblings to whom chance and murder denied an archival posterity or to count the unborn children of the murdered. This army of ghosts travel with the reader through Alfandary's story as they have travelled with him throughout his life in the "human dwelling-place". But it is possible – necessary too, if we are to live fully and the future is to exist beyond the shadow of the past – to express the "mental entity", the private jumble of images and over-determination, within the public framework of shared languages and ideas.

The "free art of psychological investigation", Zweig wrote, "often produces almost certain truths, arrived at by logical reflection". This was optimistic. In 1934, when Leon Cohen was planning his wedding, Robert Graves published *I, Claudius*. Graves combined historical erudition with philological boldness and called this the "the analeptic method — the intuitive recovery of forgotten events by a deliberate suspension of time". He believed that if a mind could be "trained to think wholly" in the mental patterns of the past, the imagination would intuitively select and arrange material from its sources and recover the truth wie es eigentlich gewessen. He happened to be Otto von Ranke's great-nephew.

Graves could close his eyes and reconstruct the ancient Roman forum in his mind's eye. Joyce joked that, if Dublin were destroyed, it could be reconstructed from *Ulysses*. He also called his novel a reconstruction of a "vanished world", the world that vanished along with much else of the old world in 1916, the year of the Somme, the Easter Rising in Dublin, and the photograph in which the entire Cohen family sit together on the steps of what we must assume is their family home in Salonica – minus Isaac, Leon's older brother, who may have been behind the camera, recording his family before the brothers' wanderings began. These are almost certain truths, arrived at by logical reflection. But they cannot be certain.

Ulysses is the Latinised name of Odysseus. The *Aeneid* records the later, Latinized adventures of Aeneas, the son of a prince and a goddess who fought the Greeks at Troy. The barrier between the present and the "vanished world" is that of war. The reconstructions of myth and memory cannot revive the dead, but they can "summon the underworld" of the not-living, as Theo Richmond did in *Konin: A Quest* (1995), his reconstruction of the world before the war. The stories that result are forms of memorial autobiography: postmemory, Rony Alfandary calls them. Recent research into the descendants of Holocaust survivors suggests that the trauma is passed on not only through the usual means – the omissions of memory, the demands to remember – but also through epigenetic changes. The postmemory of war may be printed into our DNA as well as printed in books.

The disjuncture between the external, social world and the internal, irrational drama generates *das Unheimlich*, that half-translatable term whose original German carries not just the "uncanny" sense that the familiar is foreign and the foreign familiar, but also the recognition that while we may feel we are at home in world, we are not as embedded as we might like to think. Europe's Jews were disembedded from their nations and homes in an historical instant: almost overnight, Salonica went from being the "Jerusalem of the Balkans" to a city without Jews.

We can more easily imagine the past of Salonica's Jews than the future that was denied to them by Nazi Germany and its armies of willing collaborators. Postmemory is perpetually accompanied by its double and dopplegänger, the might-have-been and might-have-lived. In recent decades, new and disembodied technologies have turned hundreds of thousands of Jews into autobiographical historians: joining genealogical websites and sending off saliva swabs to discover new materials for the narratives of memory and new genealogies of postmemory. Perhaps, this is a way of sharing the weight of history and making the unbearable more bearable. Perhaps, the dilution of sorrow and the expansion of living contacts offer a way of attaining the "ordinary unhappiness" that Freud thought a good-enough outcome of a personal reckoning with the past.

*

I end as Rony Alfandary begins, with a personal story. I was booked to speak at a literary conference in Corfu. The organizers sent the usual information: flights and hotels, panels and topics, compulsory dinners and optional excursions. One name jumped out from the list of speakers.

From childhood, I had heard that my mother's family, the Franco then Franken then Franklin family of Spanish then Dutch then German then English then American Jews, was related by marriage to a Sephardic family from somewhere in southeastern Europe via someone called Millie Alfandary. The details of this exotic association were vague, but it was asserted that one of Millie's descendants had joined the Royal Air Force. My maternal grandfather Jimmy Franklin had volunteered as an RAF pilot "before the balloon went up" in 1939 and been killed on active service in 1943. I was close to my grandmother Betty as child and would stay with her for long periods. In her guest room, Jimmy's photograph, slightly larger than life, was the last thing I saw each night before falling asleep. I was, she said, just like him.

The image of the grandfather I had never known merged with the idea of the person I might become, and in the organized way of association, the notion of an airborne Alfandary attached itself to these thoughts as a kind of supplementary confirmation. I was like Jimmy, we were like them and the flying Alfandary's voluntary service seemed to vindicate my grandfather's self-sacrifice. When I discovered that I was not a pilot material – it was all physics and maths – I felt like I had failed my grandparents and their memory. Rony Alfandary describes a similar pile-up of loss and compensatory images and fantasies in linking his middle name, Leon, with his murdered great-uncle Leon Cohen, and then "finding" the lost Leon in the form of the poet and songwriter Leonard Cohen.

Before our appointment in Corfu, Rony and I had each conducted the now-customary internet investigation into the other speakers – Google has turned us all into microhistorians of a sort. During the small talk at the conference's first session, I opened with a gambit typical between Jews, a people whose sacred texts include extensive and, if you're a historian or a new parent in search of unusual names, invaluable genealogies: "My mother's family were related to an Alfandary".

It turned out that one day in the 1980s, while Rony was working on his master's degree at the University of Nottingham, he had received a phone call from a member of this Anglo Alfandary family. They had not been able to establish a genealogical link, which is as good as almost certain truths can get these days, but neither had they concluded that they were completely unrelated. The caller had, though, mentioned serving in the RAF.

Those members of the Franken family who did not emigrate to Britain or America were deported and murdered. As with the Cohens of Salonica, a single member escaped to British-controlled Palestine in the Thirties; unlike the Cohens of Salonica, the dead left no letters to read. The same applies to my mother's maternal family, the Lincenbergs of Tarnow, Poland. The descendants of that fugitive run a guest house in the Negev Desert. Sitting in the broiling shade with my eldest daughter and our distant but uncannily close cousin Tomer, I recalled that his brother had been a pilot, killed on active service in the Yom Kippur War. I filed his image with that of my grandfather and the mystery Alfandary.

Of the branches of my father's family, the Vysovatys, sent a swamp-draining pioneer to the Land of Israel in the 1920s, but who knows what became of him. The rest, dozens and dozens of Greenbaums and Slovitches and Dreiers from Bialystok, went down into the pits or up into the air in the Holocaust. "There'll be the breaking of the ancient Western code", the other Leonard Cohen wrote in "The Future", a song that can only conceive of a future on the evidence of the past, and hence as "murder". A few years ago, a man emailed me to inform me that the Slovitches of Bialystok were related to Joseph Soloveitchik, a vital figure in the spread of Modern Orthodoxy in the United States, and were there any rabbis or intellectuals in the family? No, I said, not yet. This information, imparted to the young and impressionable, may yet fulfil the prophecy and turn the thin skein of genealogical speculation into future fact.

Who were all these people, those names on the registries of small-town births, death and marriages that the Mormons have scanned and distributed as part of their mad campaign to retroactively save lost souls, the permanently young faces on photographs of the kind that the Cohens posed for when Leon's brother Isaac was leaving for Paris? They were the cousins of my grandparents, and their children would, as second and third cousins do, have looked like my parents and me and my siblings. There are lives unlived that we cannot imagine – the lives of the kind that Rony Alfandary's grandmother charged him to remember and somehow enact – and there are the lives lived that we do not know about.

The day after visiting Tomer Lincenberg in the Negev, I took my daughter swimming on the beach at Tel Aviv. The man next to me had a son of about the same age. We looked like each other, and our children both noticed. This is not the first time this has happened to me. I gather that it's a common experience, especially among people whose present lives are imprinted by uncommon historical forces.

In 1913, when Freud finally did visit Rome, he visited the Forum, map in hand, and overlaid the images in mind. Afterwards, he sent a postcard to Karl Abraham of the Arch of Titus who celebrates the desecration of the Temple at Jerusalem and preserves the image of its menorah, a symbol of freedom. "Der Jude überlebt's", Freud wrote. "The Jew survives it".

Dr. Dominic Green is deputy editor of *The Spectator's* US
Edition and a Fellow of the Royal Historical Society.

Part 1

Introduction

Introduction

The end, the beginning and all that was left in between

The facts are stark, if little known – before World War II, the Jewish community of Thessaloniki (in its old Ottoman name – Salonica) in Greece numbered more than 50,000, the largest single ethnic minority in this Mediterranean port city which had known many past glories. When the war was over, only 5,000, less than 10%, of the Jews survived. About 45,000 people, men, women and children, were taken from the city by the local Greek police, supervised by the SS Nazi police, and between March 15th and August 10th 1942, nineteen convoys took them to their deaths in the Auschwitz concentration camp. Of the 340,000 Jews lived in France in 1940, more than 75,000 were deported to death camps, where about 72,500 were killed, about 20%.[1]

As Eva Hoffman (b. 1945), a Polish Jewish writer, wrote, the shadows of the survivors of the Holocaust continue to haunt the future generations.[2] Even though these future generations are far removed from the actual experiences of World War II, the stories told, and the stories avoided, continue to have a deep impact upon the psyches of the children and the grandchildren. They are passed on through unconscious processes, uncanny in nature, creating psychic implants in the souls of the children and grandchildren, where they continue to exert a heavy burden.

Ever since I developed a consciousness of being a part of a family, a part of a collective history, I have felt that the near annihilation of that Jewish community, and its branches elsewhere in Europe, was affecting me as if I were there myself. When my life's circumstances are examined, as I have done as part of my training and practice of psychoanalytic psychotherapy and as a writer over the last thirty-five years, I have come to the conclusion that the traces of the haunting memories I remember are not of events I have experienced myself. The events this book studies took place twenty years before I was born. They had been projected into me and have become unconsciously my own. The stories of the Holocaust that I had been exposed to since I was a child have moved me to be and act in ways it has taken me many years to make sense of. I have found that I was not just making life-choices based upon my own deliberations and options but also based upon deeper layers I was not yet aware of. It was as if I was obeying an inner dictum I could not comprehend, let alone control.

My psychoanalytic training and practice have taught me that the mental and emotional mechanism that has facilitated those processes is called, in short, *repetition compulsion*, which encompasses a wide array of mental and emotional processes.[3] It is through those insights that I have come to understand that what I thought of as haunting, traumatic memories are indeed traces of *postmemory*, that is vivid experiences and "memories" of events, which clearly did not happen to me but affect me as if they did.[4]

I have since formulated my own definition of *postmemory* which is as follows: The realization (always in retrospect) that one is being driven (in the Freudian sense of dual drive) by events that had taken place before one's actual sensual experience. One finds himself haunted by and repeating patterns of behavior, forms of relationships and (obsessive) ideas and emotions which cannot be explained solely by one's own individual history and current circumstances. It is only through an in-depth creative investigation that one can uncover the unconscious roots of the repetition one has been engaged with. Once the pattern is revealed and made conscious, it can become postmemorial work. Otherwise, if it remains unconscious, it can lead to pathological symptomatic behavior, either as an individual or as a collective.

This is a study of a memory of events that did not happen to me but have been affecting me as if they did. It tells the story of the Salonica Cohen family who have died in the Holocaust, based upon the interpretation of hundreds of letters which were discovered during the last two decades.[5] As Eli Wiesel (1928–2016) wrote, I often found myself writing so as not to lose my sanity, but often found myself only being able to write from an insane part of my awareness, as it is impossible to write about the Holocaust without losing one's sanity.[6] I hope that, as he wrote, I have been able to create a legacy of words, not so much to prevent history from repeating itself (as that would be a far too ambitious and crazy ambition), but to "simply" preserve a record of how the postmemory of the Holocaust has shaped me.

There are many such memorial stories, and this tale humbly joins them. It focuses upon the Cohen family who lived in Salonica.[7] Before World War II, the Cohens counted more than thirty: Shabtai and Rachelle Cohen, their nine children, spouses and grandchildren (Figure 1). All but one daughter, Rita, her husband Shmuel Parenti (often referred to as *Sam* in the letters) and their children died during the war, either in the concentration camps or in unknown circumstances. None has a grave one can visit.[8]

Two of the Cohen children, Leon and Isaac, moved to France during the 1920s, where they became a part of the Greek-Jewish community. The only survivor of the family, Rita, moved to Palestine during the 1930s. Both Greek and French Jewish communities were subject to mass deportation

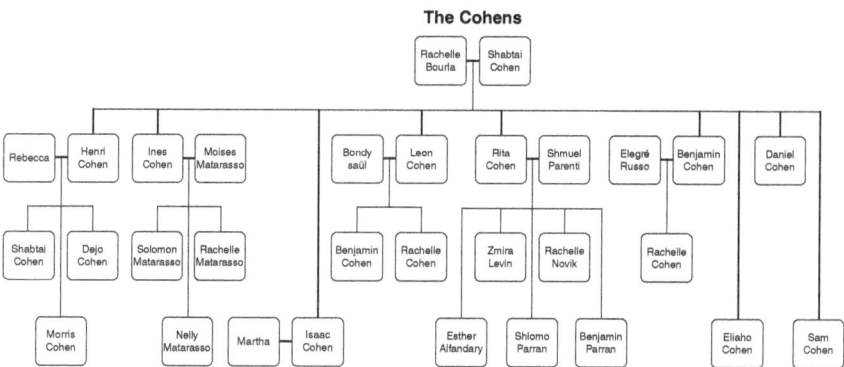

Figure 1 The Cohen Family Tree.

and murder during the 1940s by the Nazis and their local collaborators. In both Salonica and Paris, it was with the active aid of local police and municipal workers, as well as ordinary citizens, that the Jews were taken from their homes, had their properties looted and were sent to their deaths in the concentration camps.[9]

This is not a comprehensive history book of the Holocaust in Salonica or Paris. It is the story, *a microhistory*,[10] of my *postmemorial* tale of the Cohen family and in particular of Leon Cohen (1901–1942), one of the two brothers who emigrated to Paris, based upon the primary sources as found in the letters that were addressed to him and were found almost sixty years after he was murdered by the Nazis, along with his wife Bondy (Boena) (1905–1942) and their two children, Benjamin (1935–1942) and Eliane (Rachelle) (1939–1942), in Auschwitz in 1942. The exact date of their deaths is unknown. We only know when the family was deported from the Drancy transit camp on October 11th 1942, in train car number 45, as recorded by Serge Klarsfeld (Figure 2).

It is a story of a postmemory and inevitably carries the faults of a story told from a distance. And yet, it is the only possible way left to tell this story. In her seminal essay about Claude Lanzmann's Shoah, Shoshana Felman (b. 1942) wrote that being a witness is about taking responsibility for what really happened. It is about obeying the legal pledge and the juridical imperative of the oath the witness takes. It is akin to testifying before both the court of history and of the Law, in front of an audience of readers or fellow human beings. It is not just a reporting of the facts, recorded or remembered. It is an act of conjuring memory so as to present another human being and a community. Giving testimony is a moral commitment to carry on narrating history beyond its personal dimensions.[11]

The role of the testimony bearer is not one carried with ease. It is not only a burden but also a privilege. It is a burden due to the necessity of carrying

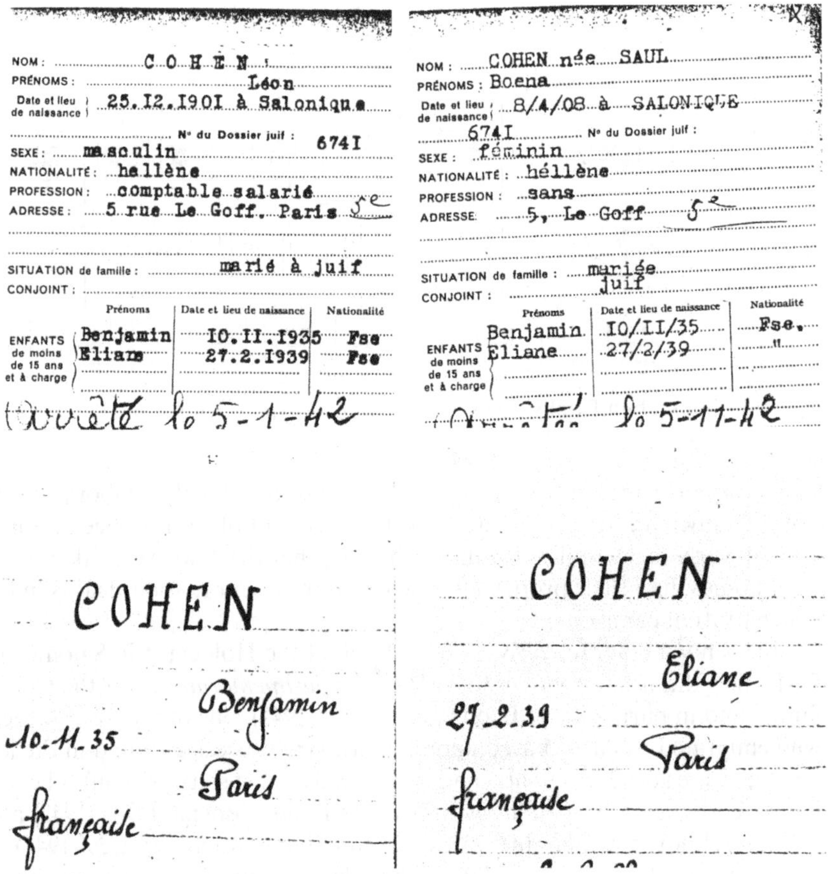

NOM : C O H E N
PRÉNOMS : Léon
Date et lieu de naissance : 25.12.1901 à Salonique
N° du Dossier juif : 6741
SEXE : masculin
NATIONALITÉ : hellène
PROFESSION : comptable salarié
ADRESSE : 5 rue Le Goff, Paris 5e
SITUATION de famille : marié à juif
CONJOINT :

ENFANTS de moins de 15 ans et à charge	Prénoms	Date et lieu de naissance	Nationalité
	Benjamin	10.11.1935	Fse
	Eliane	27.2.1939	Fse

Arrêté le 5-1-42

NOM : COHEN née SAUL
PRÉNOMS : Boena
Date et lieu de naissance : 8/4/08 à SALONIQUE
6741 N° du Dossier juif :
SEXE : féminin
NATIONALITÉ : hellène
PROFESSION : sans
ADRESSE : 5, Le Goff 5e
SITUATION de famille : mariée juif
CONJOINT :

ENFANTS de moins de 15 ans et à charge	Prénoms	Date et lieu de naissance	Nationalité
	Benjamin	10/11/35	Fse.
	Eliane	27/2/39	"

Arrêtée le 5-11-42

COHEN
Benjamin
10.11.35
Paris
française

COHEN
Eliane
27.2.39
Paris
française

Figure 2 The Cohens Deportation Cards.

it. It is a privilege as it positions the narrator along the long familial line, thus renewing and perhaps even somewhat healing a sense of continuity severed by the Holocaust. It is a possible way of combating the oblivion of forgetfulness. It is a process whereby the burden of the transmission of the traumatic memory does not turn into a haunting and crippling postmemory but lends itself to postmemorial work. In his 2019 essay on postmemory, Stephen Frosh (b. 1954) wrote that in our time, the future has collapsed. We are overwhelmed by what we have to witness. This is what haunts second and third generations – the ongoing transmission not of the experiences themselves but their dark shadows. It is an uncanny experience, both alien and deeply familiar, lying deep in the unconscious. Struggling with those shadows can be as daunting as with the concrete realities that have cast them.[12]

While Frosh and others like Hoffman wrote about the transmission of memories of Holocaust survivors to the second generation, I suggest that within the term, *second generation*, it is necessary to include future generations as well, upon whom those experiences-which-they-have-not-experienced continue to exert a meaningful and even fateful impact. A certain guilt is inherent in such a claim as it is clear that the lives and well-being of future generations are not under the immediate threat of the events of World War II, yet their shadows certainly create the sensation that those events are not in fact over and are present, like a bad dream that continues to distress the dreamer long after he had been awoken from the dream. Some of that is normally explained by the fact that caretakers transmit to their off-springs unprocessed areas of their experience and create a parental environment which is shaped by their own experience. But, somehow, in an uncanny way and yet open to psychoanalytic suggestions, the impact of those events upon those who were born after their occurrence continues to exert an influence.

It is possible to try and deny that impact and suppress its poisonous expressions or try and deal with it through interpretation and creativity. The former option can lead to pathological, individual and social consequences, while the latter can help to stop the compulsive repetition and become post-memorial work.

The Cohens' Hall of Names

This book presents the journey I have taken to turn my own potentially toxic postmemory, based upon hundreds of original documents and slivers of childhood memories, into a postmemorial project. It is my own Hall of Names. My private Hall of Names does not occupy a place in space, as does Yad Vashem's Hall of Names in Jerusalem, and it will undoubtedly draw fewer visitors from around the world, but I believe that it forms a part of the ever-increasing postmemorial Hall of Names, which the second, third and fourth generations of Holocaust survivors are creating around the world.[13]

Stepping into the Cohen family Hall of Names, I look around and see their faces. The first visual testimony is a family photo taken around 1916, where all but one member of the family are photographed together in Salonica (Figure 3).

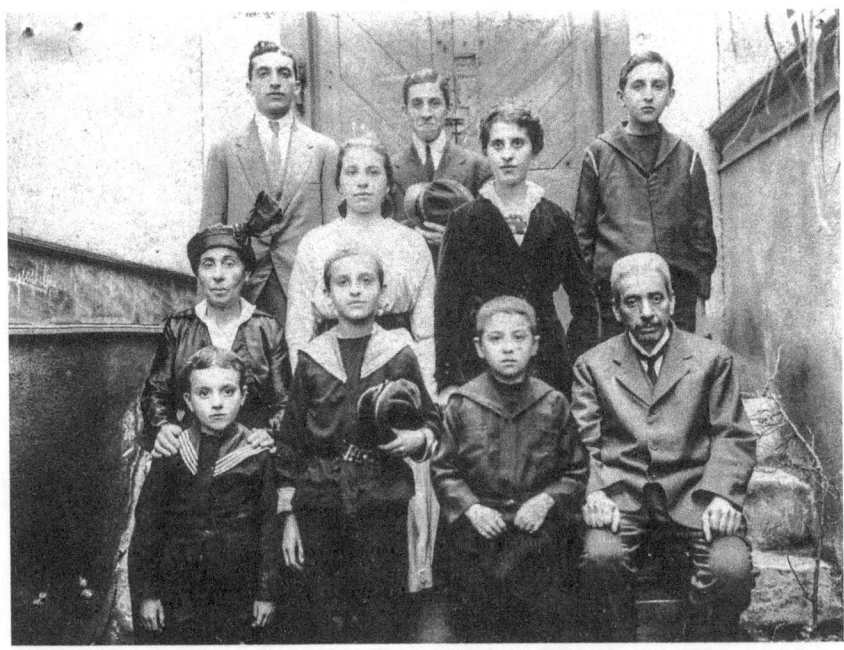

Figure 3 The Cohen Family in 1916.

They are still all together in one frame. The parents are in their late forties, while their children range from early twenties to primary school age. Eight of the nine Cohen children are present. The one missing, uncannily, is Isaac. As the story will unfold, it will become clearer that his absence from the only group photo is not so innocent.

Everybody looks serene and sombre, as is often the case in staged, formal photographs taken on some specific occasion. The exception is Leon at the back, who makes a funny face, almost a grimace, towards the photographer. There is no mention on the back of the photo as to who took it, but since it was taken before 1920 while the father of the family, Shabtai Cohen, was still alive (and judging from the approximate age of the children in the picture), it is possible that it was Isaac himself who took the photo, perhaps as a souvenir of his family before he left for France, a custom Leon was to repeat a few years later before he left himself.[14] The photo shows the family arranged in a semi-formal way, standing on the steps of what might be the entrance to their house in Salonica. Was Isaac making Leon laugh from behind the camera? Did Isaac possess a camera? It is possible. Kodak was making cameras which could be bought for about 20$ or about 100 Greek Drachma (about 290$ in today's value). It would cost a male worker the best part of a week's wage to buy such a camera in those days. Was that within Isaac's means? Considering Isaac's later adventures and a keen eye for picture postcards that he sent Leon from his trips around France, it is possible that he owned a camera then. And if he didn't, perhaps he was standing next to the photographer, making faces at the family, but only Leon responded with humour to his possible prank. The rest of the family bear serious appearances.

The head of the family, the patriarch whom we know least about, is **Shabtai** Cohen, born in 1866. He died before 1920 in unclear circumstances (Figure 4). He was apparently quite a wealthy merchant, which allowed the family to enjoy a high standard of living, including private tuition and house-keeping staff. As is seen in the picture, he also served in the Ottoman army. This picture was found in the collection and was the earliest visual testimony of his being found in the collection. His only surviving descendants, Rita's children, had never known what their grandfather looked like until a few years ago. All that ended, according to family folklore, with the financial crisis following the big fire in Salonica in 1917. *He died of a broken heart* was the sentence I had heard as a child. After his death, the family encountered on-going financial difficulties.

Shabtai married **Rachelle** Bourla, also born during the second half of the nineteenth century in Salonica.[15] As far as we know, she never worked outside her home, as expected with nine children to raise, especially after the death of her husband, who left her with young children whose private tuition still had to be paid, on top of the mounting household expenses. She was not a healthy woman but struggled throughout her life to maintain the high standard of living, including immaculate white gloves, she was accustomed to. She died in 1938 (Figure 4).

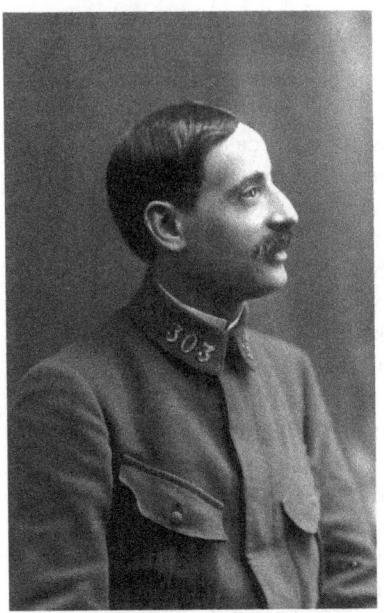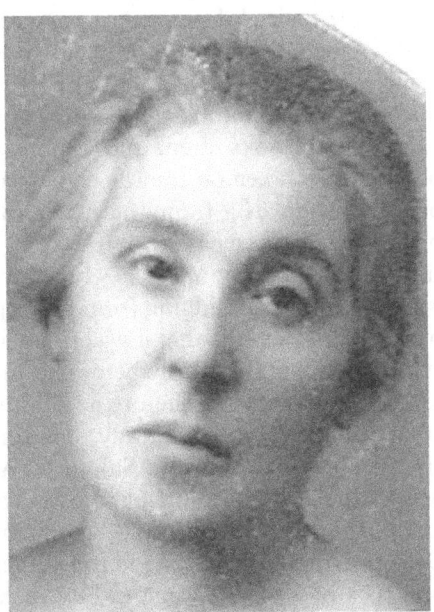

Figure 4 Shabtai and Rachelle Cohen.

Henri (Simantov) was the eldest son, born in 1893. He married Rebecca (Ricetta), also from Salonica. The couple had three children, Shabtai b. 1927, Morris b. 1930 and Dejo b. 1933. They lived in Salonica and perished in the Holocaust.

Ines (Sarah) was the second child and the eldest daughter. She was born in 1897. She married Moise Matarasso, b. 1890, also from Salonica. The couple had three children, Solomon, b. 1923, Nelly, b. 1927 and Rachelle, b. 1940. They lived in Salonica and perished in the Holocaust.

Isaac was the third child, born in 1898. He married Martha, also from Salonica but of non-Jewish origin, and they both emigrated to France in the early 1920s. They had no children and perished in the Holocaust.

Leon (Yehuda) was the fourth child, born in 1901. He married Bondy Saül, whom he met after emigrating to France. Bondy too came from an old Jewish Salonica family who emigrated to France in 1930. They had two children, Benjamin, b. 1935 and Rachelle (Eliane), b. 1939. He is the main protagonist of this memoir, since it was his letters and photos which survived him. He too perished in the Holocaust with his wife and children (Figure 5).

Rita was the fifth child and second daughter, born in 1903. She married Shmuel Parenti, also from Salonica, in 1931. They had their first child, Esther (Nina), in 1932 while still in Salonica. A year later, they emigrated to

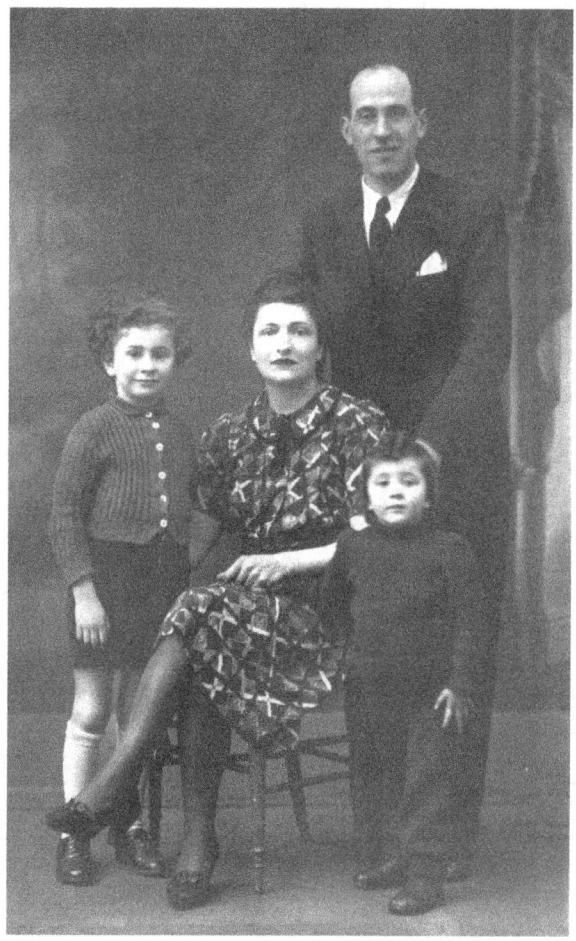

Figure 5 Leon, Bondy, Benjamin and Rachelle Cohen, circ 1942.

Palestine, where they had four more children, Zmira (Martha) 1933–2020, Shlomo (Solomon), b. 1935, and the twins Rachelle and Benjamin, b. 1939 (Benjamin died in 2012).[16] Rita and Shmuel lived in Israel until Rita died in 1986 and Shmuel in 1990. Their offspring, including 14 grandchildren and 24 great grandchildren are the only survivors of the whole Cohen.

Benjamin was the sixth child, born in 1905. He married Alegré (Simcha) Russo, also from a Jewish Salonica family. They had one child, Rachelle, b. 1934. Benjamin died from illness in 1935 in Salonica. His wife and daughter perished in the Holocaust.

Eliaho (Eli) was the seventh child, born in 1906. He did not marry. He lived in Salonica and perished in the Holocaust.

Daniel (Dino) was the eighth child, born in 1909. He did not marry. He lived in Salonica and perished in the Holocaust.

Shmuel (Sam\Sami) was the youngest child, born in 1911. He did not marry. He lived in Salonica and perished in the Holocaust (Figure 6).[17]

Looking around in the Cohen Hall of Names, two names keep recurring – Rachelle and Benjamin. Rachelle, named after the biblical figure of Rachelle, the second wife of Jacob, first appears as the matriarch of the family. She is the revered mother whose early death in 1938 caused immense grief but at the same time also spared her the horrible fate of dying in a concentration camp. As is customary in the Sephardic Jewry tradition, her name was bestowed upon other family members while she was still

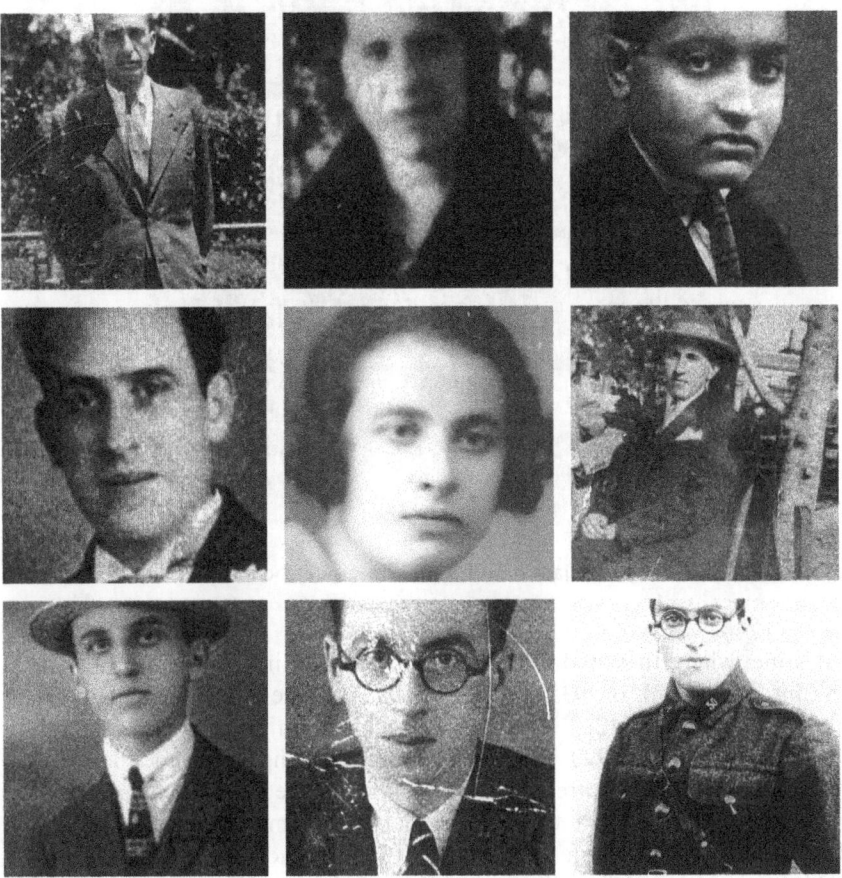

Figure 6 The Cohen Children. Top (Left to Right): Henri, Ines, Isaac. Middle: Leon, Rita, Benjamin. Bottom: Eli, Dino, Sami.

alive. And so, first, her son Benjamin's daughter, born in 1934, was given her name. And after her death, her name was given to three grandchildren: first to Leon's daughter who was born in 1939 in Paris, then to Rita's daughter born in Tel-Aviv in the same year (one of the twins), and a year later, in 1940, Ines gave birth to her third child, a daughter, who was also named Rachelle. The second recurring name, Benjamin, named after the biblical Joseph's son, first appears as Rachelle's son who died from illness in 1935 and thus too was spared the horrors of the Holocaust. First Leon in Paris named his first-born son, Benjamin, in 1935 and then Rita in Tel-Aviv named the second twin, Benjamin, in 1939. Thus, Leon's two children were named Benjamin and Rachelle and Rita's twins, the last of her five offspring, were also thus named.

The practice of the traditional naming of a child after a revered or a dead relative is indeed common and bears an uncanny significance in this story. I was given a second name after my birth: Leon. This was done with respect to my paternal grandfather, Leon Alfandary, again following a well-known Sephardic tradition on naming the first born after his paternal grandfather. But, as I grew up, I became aware that there had been another Leon in the family, but on my mother's side – Leon Cohen. Somehow, perhaps because of the name and perhaps for other reasons, my maternal grandmother, Rita Cohen, decided that I was the name bearer of her dead brother, and thus, I grew up with the strange sense of having a name that forever tied me to both branches of my family, a familial tie that often felt like a knot that I had to undo.

One clear example of the way that knot appeared in my life as a child is shown in a memory I have of when I was nine years old and visited my grandmother. After a few minutes, I noticed a French journal whose cover featured the face of the Jewish-Canadian songwriter Leonard Cohen (1934–2016). Upon seeing his name on the cover, I turned to her and exclaimed: *look, here is your brother whom you've been looking for!* All the adults in the room were amused by my confusion and mix-up of names, but I was left with a deep sense of loss, a sense that in later years developed into a deep admiration of Leonard Cohen's work, an admiration and identification that even led me to translate his first novel *Beautiful Losers* into Hebrew a few years later.

Coincidence? Childhood innocence? Perhaps. And yet, years later, I discovered another uncanny connection. In his memoir, written in 1979, my paternal grandfather, Dr. Leon Alfandary, writes about the three months he had spent in Paris during 1927, studying malaria, which had then become his area of medical specialization.[18] That was one year after the other Leon, Leon Cohen, had arrived in Paris. One of the items in the collection is Leon Cohen's diary from 1927 and on July 27th a single name is written – Alfandary. A coincidence? Perhaps, as there were other Alfandary's in Paris at the time, none of which are relatives. It is nevertheless uncanny....

Being in the Cohen Hall of Names is not just an act of remembering their faces and their stories. It is also an act of listening. It is no ordinary listening since the actual voices of the Cohens have been silenced long ago. They are no longer present in the world in any concrete way. I enter the Hall of Names, inviting you with me, to listen to the realities and silences I can recapture from the documents in the process of the creation of the patchwork of a past that never ceases to be a present for me. It is a patchwork of memories, interpretations of documents, reading of photographs, echoes of attempted recovery operations and analyses of layers upon layers of collective experience.

First, look around at the faces. These are the Cohens. Like other Jewish families in Salonica, it is likely that the Cohen family arrived at the region around the fifteenth century. They settled in the city and made a life for themselves. Until the upheavals caused by the big fire in the city in 1917 and the political turmoil that followed after the Ottoman Empire lost its grip at the beginning of the nineteenth century, I would like to assume that the Cohens were a fairly ordinary family.[19] Hard-working, mainly in commerce, maintaining the Jewish religious tradition and practice in its Sephardic form, leading simple lives occasioned by births, marriage and deaths. No great men or women came from the family, to the best of our knowledge.

The one branch of the Cohens who survived are the five children of Rita Cohen and Shmuel Parenti family Each of them led active lives, married and had children and grandchildren. The author of this memoir is a member of **the fourth generation**. Almost all of the grandchildren have married and have children (some of whom are already in their early twenties), thus creating **the fifth generation**. All in all, there are currently more than sixty individuals of this branch living in Israel and elsewhere. It boggles the mind to think how many there would have been had they not perished in the Holocaust.

They too are part of the narrative voice. All of Rita's grandchildren share stories and memories of her presence in their lives. Naturally, the older grandchildren have formed stronger links through which the transmission of the burdensome loss was passed. The younger ones have been otherwise influenced, not directly through Rita, but through their parents, her children. Each of Rita's grandchildren could have told the tale, even the youngest one, who was only six years old when she died in 1986.

The collection

The letters that this testimonial study inspired are the letters and documents found on four separate occasions and locations. They were written in four different languages: most of them are in French, some in Ladino, a few were written in Solitreo and a few legal documents are in Greek.[20] The choice of these languages, including the dominance of some, is indicative of the national and cultural complexity that the Cohen family enjoyed in Salonica, not unlike other Jewish families at that time. As Leon Saltiel wrote in his recent study of letters found in the Jewish Ghetto of Salonica, the knowledge of French showed that the family belonged to the Jewish middle class who was able to spend money on private education.[21] As will become apparent later, in times of need, such education was indeed a luxury the Cohens, like other families, had to cut.

Ladino was the language of Jews in Salonica, and other Central and Southern parts of Europe, used for more informal and daily usage.[22] It was a language acquired in transit during the expulsion of the Jewish communities from Spain in the fifteenth century. As such, it is a language of exile, travel and longing.[23]

This memoir is written in yet another language, English. Undoubtedly, some aspects of the uniqueness of the original idioms are lost through the various translations, which the scope of this study does not allow to explore properly.[24] Undoubtedly, much can be made analysing the choices that the Cohens have made in using one language or another, French being the formal language that placed them in the social and cultural position they aspired to, while Ladino was the language of home, their mother tongue, a language of idioms and playfulness, allowing them to convey messages, sometimes clandestinely, which French could not. This will have to wait for another study.

It is a Tower of Babel, a place where confusion and misunderstanding are prevalent. It is a place where multiple voices are heard simultaneously. It is also indicative of the times we live in. It is perhaps apt that such a memoir, a tale of loss and survival, will be told out of such linguistic confusion and multiplicity. As Jacques Derrida (1930–2004) wrote in his essay about

Babel, the Tower of Babel not only represents the multiplicity of language, which cannot be reduced, but it points to a defect, an inability to complete a story.[25] There will always remain a sense of incompleteness, of something missing. The familiar language contains within it an unfamiliar sound, thus evoking the Freudian sense of The Uncanny, Das unheimlich.[26] The process of translation does not aim to purely transfer meaning from one language to another in this memoir but to show the links created by the discovery and reading of the letters.

The first box was the one left behind by Rita and Shmuel in their apartment in Israel. It was kept under their bed and was taken by Rita's children after Shmuel passed away in 1990. The opening of that box was the beginning of the journey that this tale is a part of. The letters in that box were the ones Rita and Shmuel received from Rita's mother, brothers and sister from Salonica and Paris between the years 1930 and 1941. That box contained about eighty letters, handwritten in French and Ladino, as well as their envelopes and some postcards and photographs.

The physical state of those letters is often quite poor as the box went through serious physical mishaps as it was subjected to at least two floods, while the family lived in a small neighbourhood called Sova, located in the Ayalon Wadi in South Tel-Aviv during the 1930s, soon after they arrived in Palestine from Salonica.[27] Quite a few of the letters cannot be read due to their poor condition. Some of them are smudged badly. Some are torn. When the box was first opened, some of the letters had to be treated very gently. They had to be dried and pressed, which was done lovingly and with much pain by Rita's eldest daughter, Esther. Amongst them was also found a note in Ladino written by Rita, the epitaph of this book.

The box of letters was not opened immediately after Shmuel's death. The box remained unopened for a couple of years and was finally opened and examined when I asked about the addresses of the family in Salonica, as I was about to visit the city on my journey through Europe in 1993, a journey that began in Berlin and ended in Greece, while *en route* I visited, amongst other places, the Auschwitz concentration camp.

Once the box was opened, things began rolling fast. The Salonica addresses from which letters were sent during the war years were located and visited both by me and in following years by other members of the family. None of the original buildings survived. What was more significant was that the opening of the box ignited a dormant hope in Rita's children that perhaps someone from the family had survived. They knew that their father had spent many efforts trying to locate surviving family members during the 1940s and 1950s, as many other Jewish immigrants from Europe did in those years. It was not only Rita's family that he was looking for but his own uncles, aunts and cousins who too stayed in Salonica, who he eventually found out did not survive. He was unable to find a single soul but did the least he could – register their names with Yad Vashem in 1957. After he ceased searching, his children did not continue his efforts. But then, in 1993, as they looked through the letters in the box, the addresses in Paris from which Leon sent his letters captured their attention. Especially the last address: 5 Rue le Goff. Rita's children began investigating. The beginning of the search was akin to looking for a needle in a haystack. But through hard work, much perseverance and some good luck, a lead was found. Benjamin's wife, Elly, and Esther's friend, Ines Cohen (no relation), came across a photograph of Leon and Bondy in a publication by Serge Klarsfeld (b. 1935). They were able to contact Serge and his wife, Beate, (b. 1939) who provided them with the name of the person who gave them that photograph, Mireille Florent Saül from Paris. It took some very intensive overseas telephone conversations with the French telephone company until Mireille was indeed found. In a very emotional telephone conversation, it was confirmed that she was the daughter of Leon Cohen's wife's sister, Rosette (Rosa) Saül, who lived in Provence.

Even though the Saül family was only linked to the Cohens by marriage, it was the closest they got to find a lost relative. At first, it appeared that Rosette was not too keen to share information regarding what Leon and her sister Bondy may have left behind in that flat.[28]

Thanks to Mireille's insistence, the **second box** of letters was soon "found" amongst Rosette's possessions. The box had been kept, apparently, in the flat in 5 Rue le Goff soon after the war and was there for nearly two decades, while Rosa's and Bondy's brother, Edmond, lived in it.

It was only after Edmond left the flat during the late 1950s that the box was given to Rosette and kept at her home in Provence.

That box of letters contained nearly 100 letters and postcards received by Leon Cohen, first as a single man and then as a married man between 1931 and 1941. These were letters he received from his mother, his sister Ines, his brothers who stayed in Salonica, from his older brother Isaac, whom he followed to France, and from his sister, Rita, in Palestine. The flow of letters from this box stopped in 1941.

The third box of letters and documents was discovered, again "accidentally" in the same house in Provence in 2014 by Rosa, and contains about eighty letters, seventy postcards and about fifty photographs received by Leon Cohen from his mother and siblings in Salonica, Paris and Palestine between 1927 and 1940 and contains letters and documents Leon took with him to Paris after he left Salonica (Figure 7).

The discovery of **the fourth box**, early in 2017, was even a bigger surprise (Figure 8). It contained more about 100 letters, 100 photographs, 150 postcards as well as many other items such as Leon's business stamp, diary, cheque book, various legal documents, visiting cards, two small paintings done by an unknown artist and other objects, covering the period between

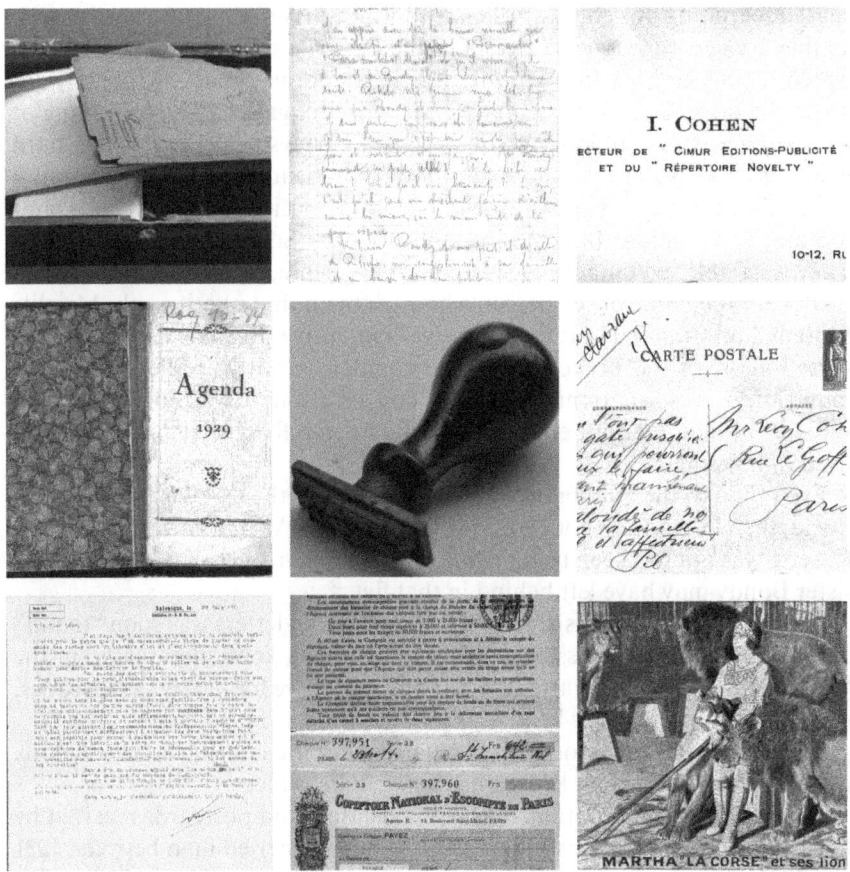

Figure 7 Items from the Third Box.

1917 and 1931. It was apparently found in the same house in Provence, but for some reason it was only announced recently. All attempts by the author and others to understand how that was possible were met with non-descript answers, ranging from '*there was a big mess when we moved*' to a simple '*I just don't know. I just found it*'. It is most tempting to speculate about the real and deeper layers of such a denial, but as it was felt that this was a sensitive issue, perhaps covering a family secret, and risked causing unnecessary hurt, it had been dropped for the time being, leaving much to wonder about. What is the story behind the gradual revelation of the boxes? What secret narratives lie beyond?

And so today, the collection contains about 400 letters, both family letters and business letters relating to Leon Cohen's occupation as an accountant in France, more than 200 postcards showing mostly Leon and Bondy's travels in France before the war and over 200 photographs, quite

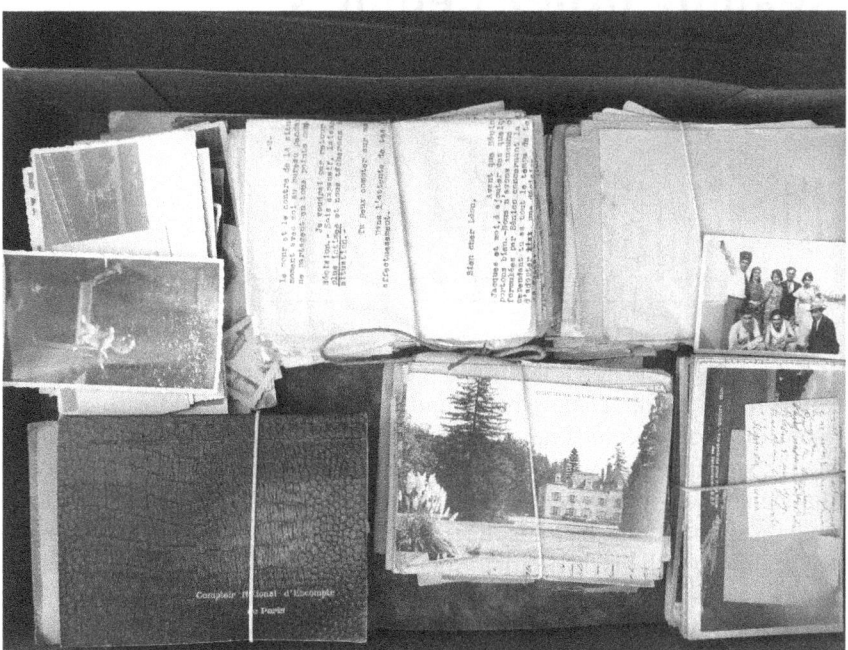

Figure 8 The Fourth Box.

a few of recognizable family members but mainly of people whose identity remains unknown to date, as well as many other times.

Overall, the Cohen collection holds more than 800 items allowing more than a glimpse into the life of Leon Cohen and his family. There are many possible narratives that can be reconstructed from the collection: the personal exchange between Leon and his siblings and mother; the professional letters exchanged with his business associates; the pictorial narratives depicted through the postcards showing Leon and Isaac's travels in France during the happy years preceding the war; the pictorial narrative told through the photographs kept in the collection, including the many photographs where unidentified people are documented; the narrative of the various artefacts found in the boxes. All these narratives will be touched upon in this book but in no way will be subjected to exhaustive analysis. That will have to be left for future research.

Reading other people's letters

When a person sits down in his room to write a letter, with the exception of letters to the editor of a newspaper and such, he is usually addressing his private words to a specific reader. He is having a dialogue through the written media, which he may well have meant to conduct verbally and directly with that person, but for a variety of reasons, prosaic or not, he writes them down on paper. Once done, he folds the paper and places it inside an envelope, often sealing it with his own saliva, sticks a stamp on it, walks down the street to the nearest post box, slips it inside and then returns home to begin the period of waiting for a reply.

The study I am writing is based upon reading and analysing letters that were written and addressed to people who are no longer alive. They cannot give their consent or deny it. All I have in terms of permission is Rita's will to remember her siblings and tell their story. It is more than a consent, it is an injunction, but only written by one protagonist in this tale.

Reading and interpreting the Cohen letters is, therefore, undertaken with a sense of caution and respect for the dead but also with a nagging sense of duty and debt. It is a sensitive material not just because of its content but due to its mere existence. Each reading enfolds within it unknown dimensions, resounding and sending echoes within one's psyche. Reading the material evokes a sense of loss and trauma. Rita's youngest son, the late Benjamin, my uncle, had told me that while compiling the first edition of the letters, based upon two boxes, tears would often well up in him, causing him to take frequent breaks, rush to the kitchen for a drink of cold water.[29] It was only when I was getting deeper and deeper into the writing of this book that I found myself in a very similar situation.

Overshadowing the reading of the Cohen letters is a cloud of uncertainty. One could say that Leon Cohen was fortunate enough (a sardonic use of the word) to have fragments of his life documented, allowing some kind of reconstruction and regaining of memory. What about the lives of his brothers and sister, their spouses and children, who perished in the Holocaust, leaving no material trace behind them? Whatever happened to the letters they wrote and received? To their family photos? Will they be discovered miraculously one day? More likely than not, those physical traces are lost for good and will never be recovered. All that is left of them are the traces they had left in Leon Cohen's life. These are paths this memoir is attempting to uncover and follow. Human history is often based upon the archaeological findings that are unearthed in various sites. But what about all that archaeology has not been able to find, all the material objects that have left no trace whatsoever? Who guarantees that what had survived the erosive passage of time is indeed more significant than what had perished and totally disappeared? Many histories have evaporated into thin air. History is written based upon shreds and figments. As Stefan Zweig (1881–1942) wrote in his book on Marie Antoinette in 1938, the absence of hard data in the unravelling of history leads the writer to rely upon the free art of psychological investigation, which often produces almost certain truths, arrived at by logical reflection.[30] That psychological investigation needs to be conducted with caution and perhaps even a sense of scepticism, as suggested by the English historian Robin George Collingwood (1889–1943), since what we see as history is a transcription of given narratives, which always need to be further interpreted and researched, viewing the process itself as the main source of data.[31]

The fragmented history that I have sewn together in the following pages is based upon the letters written by and to several people, mostly members of the Cohen family, and therefore does not present a single and cohesive narrative, and in more than one way represents an enactment of the past. I was not intent upon uncovering some objective truth but rather to subjectively represent what I thought had happened in the lives of my protagonists, to show the broken and fragmented vision of the life they led during those twenty years the tale covers.

The gaps are wider than the actual content. We shall have to listen to the silences as well as to the material evidence. As all the letters that were received by the family in Salonica from Palestine and Paris were lost, we are left with a very partial picture. This triangular correspondence is forever missing one of its vertices. We can only imagine the lost vertex.

The complex consideration of the treatment of the letters does not end there. Even though the authors of the letters are long dead, the present readers of the letters will be able to detect *a textual author*, as if the characters writing the letters are indeed speaking. Reading about the Cohens' lives conjures up the reality in which they lived. Questions regarding the veracity of the letters come rushing in too: is this how it *really* happened? Are the texts of the letters revealing the real circumstances of the time or are they hiding something behind? Does the reality described in them represent *an absolute truth* or an approximate truth?

The texts of the letters are not just presented as they were written. They are not just funnelled to the reader. The texts are inevitably my interpretation of them, even though I took the utmost care in their translation and the editing that was required at times.

In the spirit of the French philosopher, Michel de Montaigne (1533–1592), what will be presented in the following chapters is my *understanding* of the letters, an understanding of a sorrow too great to be expressed in a tangible emotion. He wrote that he wishes to be viewed in his own genuine, simple, and ordinary manner, without study and artifice: as it is himself that he portrays. His defects are to be read as part of his natural form.[32]

Clearly, a great distance stood between me and the letters. There is the obvious linguistic distance – the letters were written in a language that is foreign to me. They describe cultural circumstances I can only imagine and at a period almost a century ago. I am holding the letters in my hand, so I know they are real. They certainly impact and move me in tangible ways. They are concrete objects that testify to the geographical distance they travelled, as letters do. And yet, despite the linguistic, temporal and cultural distance, I hope that my understanding of the letters has been able to bridge those distances and convey the deep *intimacy* I experienced while bringing them together into this narrative, this tale of a postmemory. Like Montaigne, who had lost five of his six children in early infancy, I hope that the sharing of the tale will allow the release of the stupor that the horror of those days can impose and will allow the healing process to continue.

Key figures in the story

Who are the more significant narrative voices in this tale? To whom is it right that attention will be drawn? Is it necessary to point to particular figures, at the expense of others, in order to make it a better story? Using such literary ploys seems almost inappropriate when dealing with such subject matter, and yet, these considerations are also inevitable. Decisions need to be made, and it is better if they are made out in the open. There's a story to be told, and it needs to be told in the best possible way.

There are four key figures that are prominent in the letters: Leon Cohen in Paris, who is the recipient of the majority of letters, his older brother Isaac, their sisters Ines in Salonica and Rita in Tel Aviv.

The other five Cohen brothers and their mother, Rachelle, as well as other characters such as spouses and acquaintances, are there too but will only be mentioned if pertinent to the key figures themselves. The father of the family, Shabtai Cohen, who had been a wealthy merchant in Salonica, died at a relatively young age. This would also explain the moving away of Isaac and Leon to Paris in search of financial security and stability. The widow, Rachelle, relied upon her children to support her. And they did.

The first personal letter sent to Leon after he had moved to Paris is from his younger brother, Eli, in Salonica and is dated January 22th 1925. The letter is written on the back of a photograph of Ines' oldest son, Solomon.

I'm sending you a postcard of the cute Solomon [Figure 9]. He seemed to be annoyed. I have received two letters from you, including the content in the envelopes (Money?).[33] *I'll reply in more length tomorrow. We are very happy that you are progressing in your work and becoming more independent.*

At home everyone is fine. As in Marseilles, the weather is very good and it hardly feels like winter. We received a postcard from Isaac and also still waiting for a letter from him.

Yours,
Eli

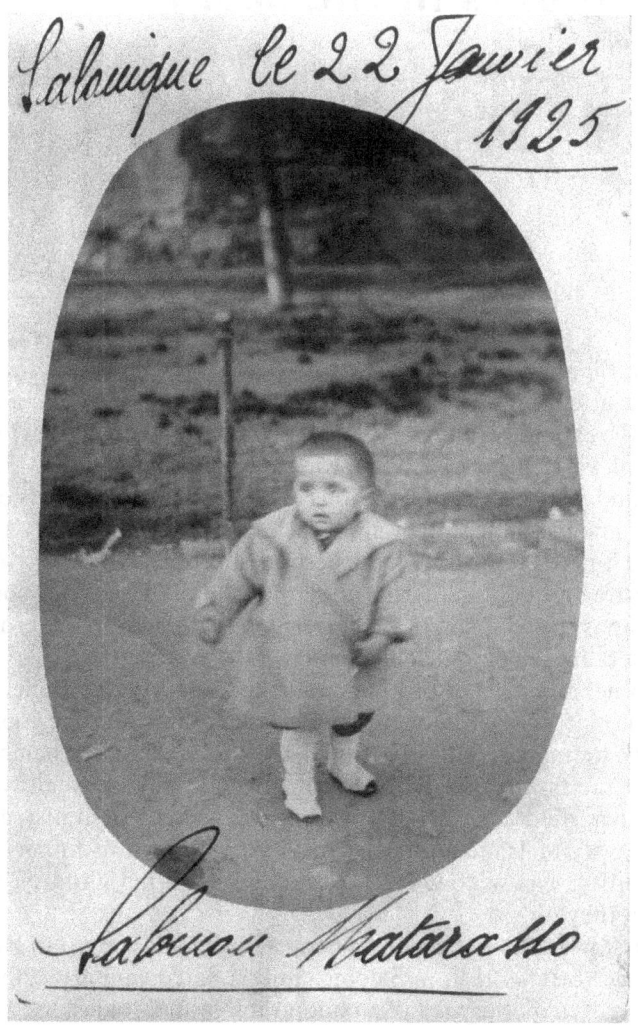

Figure 9 Solomon Matarasso 1925.

The first letter that was written by Leon himself is addressed to Shmuel Parenti in Salonica, who is about to marry Leon's sister, Rita, and is dated October 14th 1930.

Dear Sam,

Allow me to address you in such an intimate way even before I can call you my dear brother-in-law? Is it necessary to greet you? Is it necessary to compliment you on your choice of a bride? I will only say that I wish you much happiness and a long life. I am beginning to grasp that that is true happiness: home, a loving, beautiful, clever, loyal and good-natured wife, one of us.

After one is married to such a woman, one can face life with more courage. I will be brief today and hope that you respond quickly so that we can get better acquainted. My brother Isaac also sends his greeting. He and his wife Martha are always busy. Even I only see him once or twice a week here in Paris, and even that only briefly.

Yours,
Leon

The wedding took place in Salonica on March 11th 1931. The young couple would soon leave Greece and settle in Palestine. Young Shmuel Parenti was a Zionist activist. He was elected by the Zionist Federation of Greece to be a member of the organizing committee appointed to arrange for the 8th Greek Zionist Congress.[34] This was based upon his local activity in the Zion Flag (*Degel Sion*), a Salonica Zionist Association, which included being the Treasurer of the local Jewish Zionist football team (Figure 10). Parenti was elected in 1930 by the Zionist Federation to be a member of the Hirsch Quarter committee, a local Jewish group in charge of local Jewish affairs in that district that was predominately Jewish. It was the very same district where years later, the Jews of Salonica were rounded up before being sent to their deaths in Auschwitz.[35]

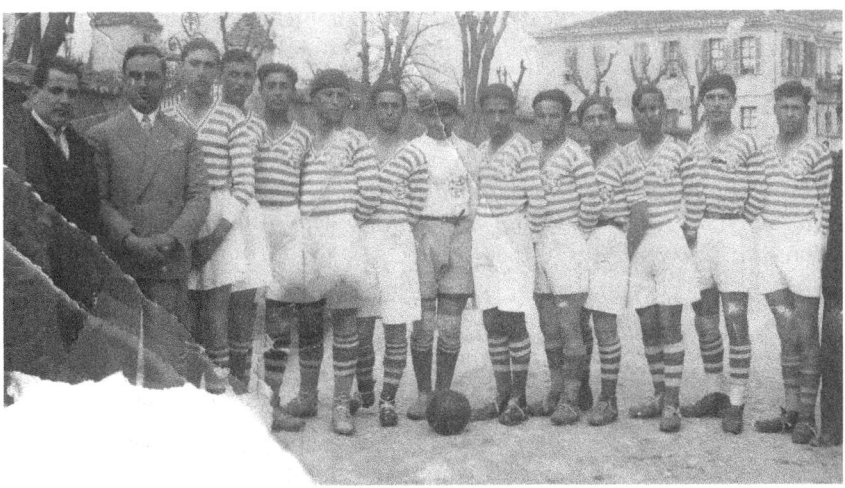

Figure 10 Shmuel Parenti & Jewish Salonica FC 1930.

The last letter in the collection is a letter sent to Bondy's sister, Rosette. It is dated November 16th 1942 and needs no explanation.

Melle Denise Ertzlichoff to Paul and Rosette Paris, Wednesday, November 16th 1942

... The concierge from 5 rue Le Goff has asked me to say she would very much like to have news as she liked your sister dearly... As you have heard, I was at the Broussais hospital where I had been since October and from which I came out last week. I was being treated for arthritis of the upper foot and bone decalcification. You probably heard these details from your sister Bondy as she came to see me on November 2^d with the two little ones on her way to put flowers on her uncle's grave...So when Melle Froment (The concierge) *came to tell me the dreadful news, how they were all arrested, your poor sister, your brother-in-law, the two little ones, your dear parents, your sister Suzanne, I could not believe in such a terrible misfortune.*

Is it possible such things can be done, taking young men away is one thing, we are at war, but women, poor little children and elderly people, it is too horrible, especially in the way the concierge from 5 rue Le Goff described it, it is unthinkable and so appalling, your poor sister crashing down on the floorboards with eyes of dread, I am so worried about her health and above all little Benjamin and little Elaine, if they had at least been left with you, or with me, I would have taken care of them and I am sure she would have felt easier knowing them to be safe.

I was told that the friend across from them got a letter in November telling him they were at Drancy, but were going away that very evening to where they did not know.

Maybe you have some news as I heard you were left free though I cannot believe this arrest is about religion, I suppose it is to do with them being Turkish citizens, as I read in the papers about Turkey siding with England and Russia. They should have gone away early in November for I know many who are safe and well in Lyon and Marseille.

I should very much have liked to come to see you and talk in person about all these sad things but I cannot walk and am still in the same state regarding my foot which gives me a lot of pain, and then I worry so much about your sister and the two poor children, they were so sweet.

If you have any news, I beg of you dear Mme Rosette let me know, or if you can come to see me it would make me so happy; hoping you will come – please pass on my regards to your husband...

Denise

Almost twenty years had passed between the first letter in 1923 and the last one in 1942. During that time, around 400 letters were exchanged. Of those, only nineteen were written by Leon himself. It is not possible to do justice to the amount and details of the information and emotions exchanged in these letters within the scope of this introductory chapter. They are brought here, quoted in full, as an indication of the drama and tragedy that unfolded.

As mentioned before, most of the letters in the collection were those received by Leon Cohen in Paris, who is the main protagonist in this tale. At first, during the twenties, they describe a young man working as an accountant, first in Paris, then in Marseilles and then back in Paris. After some quite considerable difficulties during the first few years, including a failed business venture with his brother, he seemed to have done well for himself and managed to stay in business as a free-lance accountant during the economic turbulence of those years. He maintained close ties with friends from Salonica, who also served as a network both socially and professionally. He was, like many people at that time, an *émigré*, finding a home away from home within the Greek immigrant community in Paris, which was a very cosmopolitan, cultured and lively city during the *roaring twenties* and thirties.[36] The contents of some of these letters are very jovial and show strong friendly connections between young men who enjoy their years as popular single men, seeking fun in their personal lives and promotion in their professional lives.

Later, in the mid-1930s, Leon married Bondy Saül, herself from a family of Salonica Jews, who had emigrated to France.[37] That is an occasion for much celebration and greetings. The letters from that period describe domestic happiness as well as longing for the families back home. Interwoven in the letters are hopes that the Cohen family will reunite. Leon expressly hopes that his brothers, sister and mother join him in Paris. He even hopes for his sister in Palestine to come and join him with her family, even though he acknowledges that the life they have made in the growing Jewish community there binds them to that remote land. In reality, after he left Salonica in 1925, Leon Cohen never again saw his Salonica family nor his sister in Palestine.

Once married, Leon and Bondy seemed to lead a relatively comfortable family life in Paris. Leon is doing well in his business as a free-lance accountant. Dozens of postcards from their trips in France attest to that. In many photographs, they are shown to be enjoying the countryside, the sea and friendly encounters. Soon, they have two young children, Benjamin, born in 1935 and Rachelle, born in 1939. The collection contains many photographs of the couple and their children as well as postcards collected during their trips in France in those happy years (Figure 11).

Many of the letters Leon received were from his older brother, Isaac, and his Christian wife, Martha (Figure 12). The figure of Isaac is a dark one. What Isaac did for a living during those years remains somewhat of

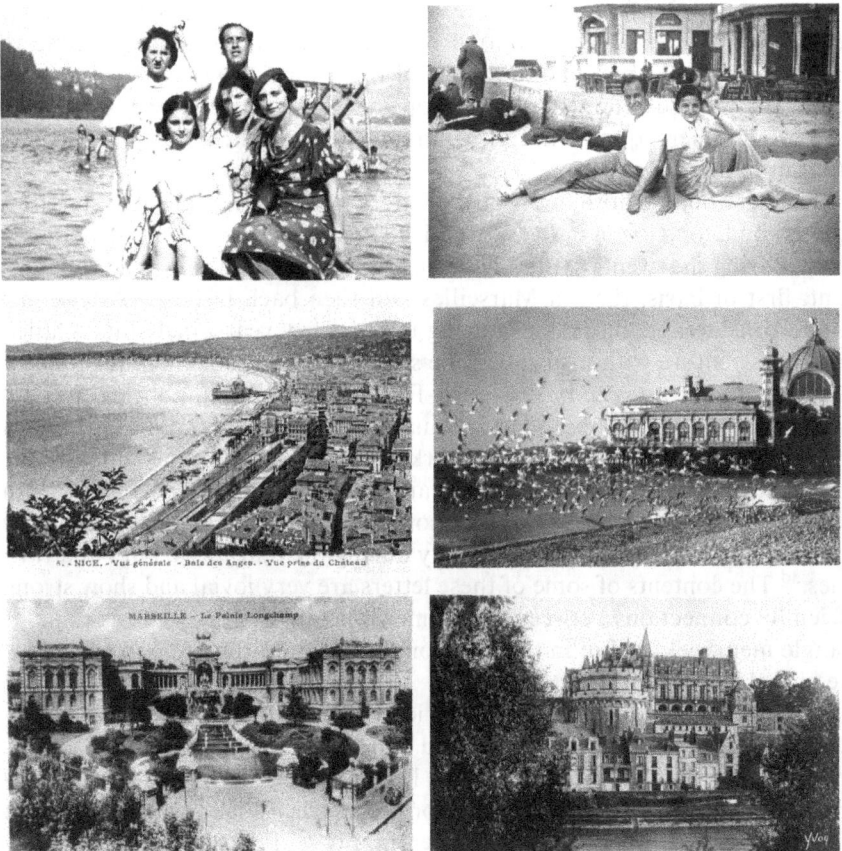

Figure 11 Leon and Bondy Travelling.

a mystery. He was involved in various commercial activities, including attempts at starting a restaurant. Some of these activities involved export and import. What is clear is that, mostly, he did not fare well in business and was often in debt and, more than once, on the run from debtors. On more than one occasion, he had to leave Paris or at least to pretend that he was leaving Paris in an attempt to avoid his debtors. It seems that the couple did not have any children, at least not while the correspondence was taking place. Isaac seldom wrote letters that did not contain requests for financial assistance. His brothers, sisters and mother often reproached him for not keeping in touch. When he did, it was only to ask for more money or to boast of a new venture he was sure was going to turn into a huge success. He seemed to vacillate between excesses: either deep in sombre moods, prepared even to sell his wife's dowry to rescue himself, or else at times of apparent success, taking lavish holidays in France and sending postcards from his tours. His whereabouts during the war or the question of what actually happened to him remained unresolved to this day. Numerous archival and online searches, including Beate and Serge Klarsfeld's book which documented the lists of Jews taken from France to concentration camps, revealed no evidence of his fate. That list does include the names of Leon, Bondy Cohen and their children as being inboard train convoy no. 45, which took them to their death in Auschwitz but does not contain any reference to Isaac. There is a reference to an Isaac Cohen born in Salonica who was on that very same convoy to Auschwitz, but his year of birth is given as 1896, so it remains an open case as to whether that was the same Isaac.[38] During the writing of this book, another attempt to gather information was also made through the *French Commission for the Compensation of Victims of Spoliation Resulting from the Anti-Semitic Legislation in Force during the Occupation,* a

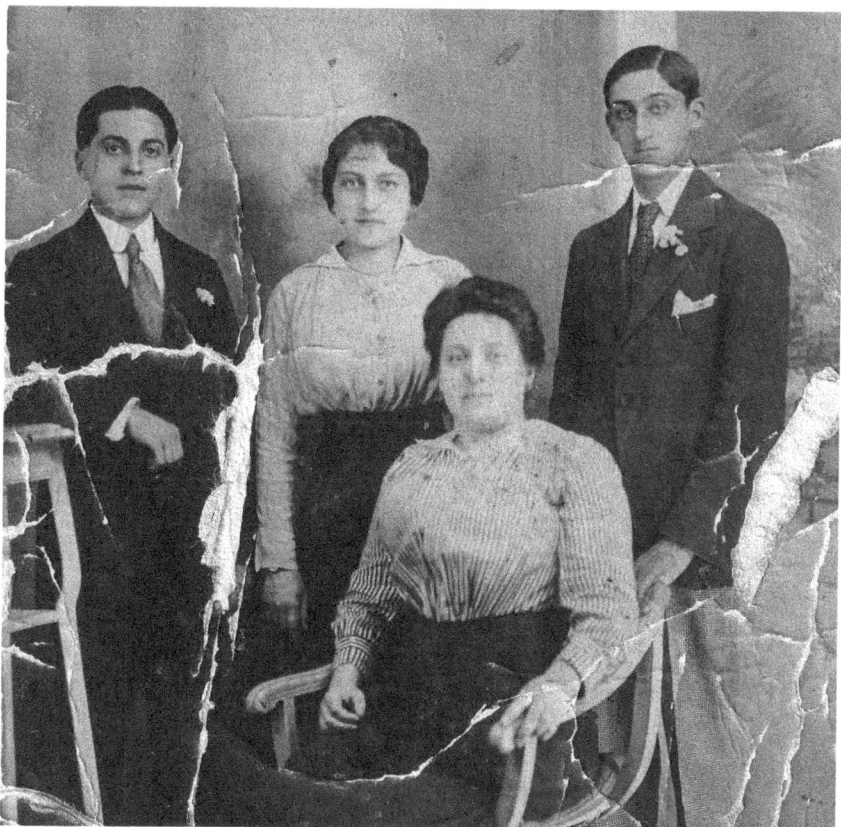

Figure 12 Isaac & Martha Cohen and Martha's Mother & Brother 1925.

governmental agency established by the French President Jacques Chirac in 2000, but so far have not yielded any results.

The figure of Ines Cohen is portrayed as the loving, benevolent and caring elder sister. She was married to Moise Matarasso and was the mother of three children (Figure 13). It was Ines who was Rachelle Cohen's main source of comfort in the difficult years. She remained near her mother and, in fact, took her into her household. She led a relatively stable family life with her husband and three children and was the backbone of the Cohen family in Salonica. It was to her that Leon turned when in need. It was from her that the maverick Isaac shied away, fearing her disapproval. It was with her that Rita conducted the most moving exchanges through letters. Like her mother, she had to deal with health issues, which were becoming increasingly hard to manage as the economic situation in Salonica worsened. In her letters, she comes over as an honest and direct woman, stern but also empathic when she realised that it was expected of her. In the letters she wrote to her brother in Paris and her sister in Tel-Aviv, she always made an effort to keep them updated with the goings-on in her family. Apart from informing them of her children's achievements, such as success in their studies or reaching Bar-Mitzva age, she was always concerned with her younger siblings' future. The main goal, common to many Jewish families, was to see that they got married into good families as well as having good jobs that would allow them to provide for their future spouses and children. As will unfold in later chapters, despite her efforts, events did not always happen as she had wished them to. Ines, her husband and his parents and siblings, as well as their three children, were sent to the concentration camps like the vast majority of Salonica Jewry in 1943. No trace was found of their burial place. It was my mother's hope that they had all died along the torturous journey to the camps and did not have to undergo the painful existence there, as was written about in many survivors' testimonies, the most famous of which was Primo Levi's (1919–1987) *If this is a man*, where he recounts encounters with Salonica Jews, whom he described as the toughest of all inmates.[39]

The fourth figure, Rita Cohen, my grandmother, was the fifth child. She was an independent woman who worked as a teacher in the *Alliance Israélite Universelle* in Salonica.[40] She did not hurry to enter into a matrimonial bond and married relatively late when she was already thirty years old, which was quite unusual for a woman in those times and was usually attributed to her having some disqualifying characteristics. That was not apparently the case with her. She simply did not want to compromise and apparently had been in a relationship with a colleague at school, which her family did not approve of.[41] She was eventually married off to Shmuel Parenti, who was a journalist and a Zionist activist and was introduced to her by her beloved brother Benjamin who knew him through their mutual work at the Theodor Herzl Association in Salonica.[42] The two were married in 1930. Rita became

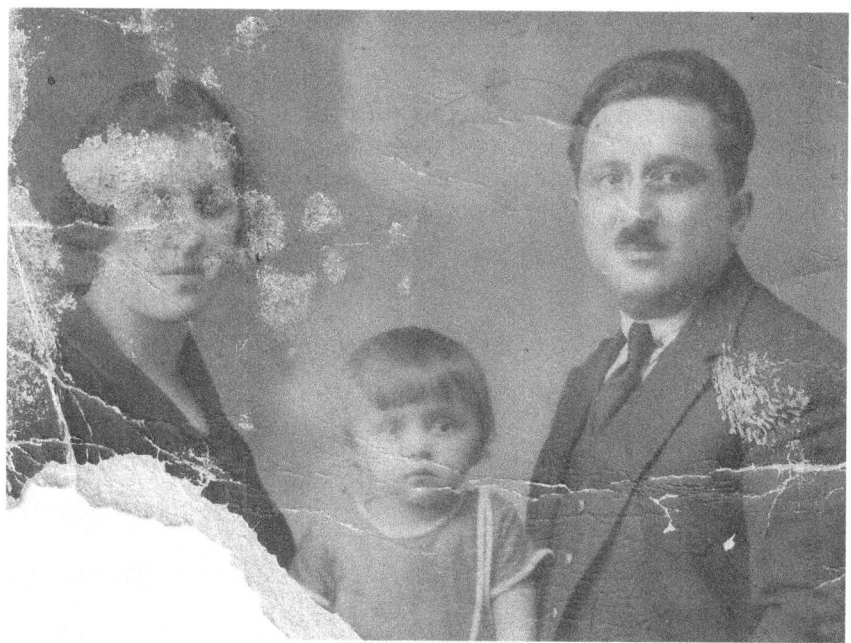

Figure 13 Ines, Moise & Solomon Matarasso.

pregnant soon after and gave birth to their first of five children, Esther, in 1932. Shmuel had made very clear from the beginning his intentions to fulfil his Zionist goal and emigrate to Palestine, and despite her reluctance, the young couple and their child (Rita was also pregnant with their second child) made their way by boat to Jaffa in 1933. As the letters sent to Salonica from Tel-Aviv in the following years showed, those were very hard times. Rita gave birth to four more children, including twins, and had to live at a much lower standard of living she was accustomed to. Like many immigrants, Shmuel had to take on menial work and could not continue his original occupation as a journalist. Eventually, he managed to open a stall at the Carmel Market in Tel-Aviv and was able to provide for his children, all of whom were able to acquire a respectable profession, marry and have children through his support. The two maintained a humble way of life but provided a safe and loving home for their five children during the tough pre-state years in Israel, going through the many riots that preceded the establishment of the state. This particular tale ended in 1942, but this branch of the Cohens lives on, the only survivors of the Salonica Cohen family. I have grown up with the assertion that it was thanks to my grandfather's Zionism that we all had a life to live. And at the same time, I was aware that Rita maintained a longing for the life she had left behind in Salonica in order to follow her husband's ambitions. Since she was not herself a Zionist, it was clear that she had often regretted that move but was torn by the knowledge that had she not made it, her fate would have been like her siblings' – death in the concentration camps. After she parted from her mother, sister and brothers in 1933, she never saw them again. That was her constant sorrow, a sorrow that she projected onto future generations, a sorrow that had developed into my sense of being a living monument for all she had lost. A memory of her loss had developed into my postmemory.

Making choices

One of the issues that resound through the reading of the letters is the question regarding the choices that were made. Did Leon Cohen know what was facing him and his family? Can traces be found in the letters demonstrating that he struggled with choices, moral and practical, that determined the fate of his family? The reading of the letters is inevitably tied up with the sense and even the wish that the course of events could have been differently conducted. If only Leon Cohen had read the signs in a similar way to his brother-in-law Shmuel Parenti, perhaps, he would have moved from Paris in time and thus saved himself and his family.

When asked by Theodore Reik (1988–1969), his disciple, how to make a major choice in one's life, Sigmund Freud (1856–1939) replied during the early twenties that judging by his own experience, such decisions could only be found in the unconscious, that deep layer within ourselves. In such cases, we should allow ourselves be governed by the deepest place in our psyche.[43]

In the French book *un Sac de Billes*, based upon the memoir of the Holocaust survivor Joseph Joffo (1931–2018), the narrator recalls the life-changing decision his father made in 1941 after the Nazis occupied Paris.[44] Promising seven-year-old Joseph and his twelve-year-old brother Maurice that he will follow soon with the rest of the family, he urges them to leave home that night with very few belongings, some money and an instruction sheet they must destroy. The boys managed to escape and reach the Free Zone where they underwent a series of dramatic events, including a capture by the Nazis from which they escaped through their ingenuity and the kindness of a Protestant priest. When they were eventually reunited with their family in Paris at the end of the war, they found that their father, who set them free by letting them go, himself did not fare well and perished in a concentration camp.

It is possible to think of the choice he made that night came from that deep place Freud referred to upon giving Reik his advice. It was a choice that saved their lives.

Was Leon Cohen faced with a similar situation when realizing that the Nazi presence in Paris was not going to ease up? He too was leading a fairly comfortable life up to the Nazi invasion. As a successful independent accountant, he was able to provide well for his young family. Moreover, he was doing well enough in those years, which followed much harder periods when he first arrived in Paris, still a bachelor, in 1925, to send money back home to his family in Salonica. This is also attested by his residency in the sixth Arrondissement, near Jardin de Luxembourg and the family vacations in the countryside.

From what perspective is it possible to address such a question? Is it even ethical to address such a question regarding Leon Cohen's inner working? What data would be required to enable the ethical writer to even arrive at such an analysis?

Turning again back to Reik's words, one can safely repeat Freud's advice to make such choices only on the basis of self-observation and self-analysis. An individual cannot rely upon someone else's experience, even if it means repeating the same mistake time and time again. It is only after repeating the same mistake that the individual is ready to make the right choice.[45]

The questions I ask regarding the ethical aspects of reading, analyzing and writing about the letters are questions only I can answer and be accountable for. Is there ever enough temporal, spatial, emotional and intellectual perspective from which to write about such experiences as Reik suggests? I doubt it. The stories that unfold from the letters are stories that will hold within them never-ending expanding qualities, rendering any completion and therefore any appropriate perspective impossible and unattainable.

In my account, the city is an important protagonist. The presence of the city in the lives of the people inhabiting it is far greater than the place where they reside, where they walk the streets and where they lead their lives. Be it their city of origin where they feel at home or be it a foreign city to which they have exiled themselves, their story is the story of the city. The city is a transcendental entity that shapes the individual's consciousness and interacts with his unconscious. As Gaston Bachelard (1884–1962) wrote, understanding the city helps us to understand the individual and vice versa.[46] The city is not only a concrete place that can serve as a home but also a transitional dream space that can function as an asylum from unwanted external circumstances as well as repressed mental content.

As a transitional space, used in the sense Donald W. Winnicott (1896–1971), the British psychoanalyst, referred to, it can encourage creativity and play. But for that to happen, the city needs to be a mother/father figure that the individual can trust. As long as the city remains a good-enough parent, the individual can thrive and develop. Once the city becomes toxic and hostile, the individual can soon fear for their life.[47]

Unfortunately, the cities of Paris and Salonica, as well as other European cities of that time, became toxic for their Jewish inhabitants. They both offered little protection and eventually expelled the majority of the Jewish communities. The only relatively safe city for Jews in this tale was Tel-Aviv, which itself was fraught in those years in the struggle for independence and was continually threatened by the Arab resistance to the new Jewish settlement on the one hand and the British Mandate on the other hand.[48]

Postmemory and family trauma

The narratives of the twenty years contain many stories. Weddings were announced and annulled, and illnesses and deaths were recounted. Financial difficulties. Longing and admonitions that not enough letters were arriving. Those were the days when letters were the only means of communication with people across the sea or even at a shorter distance. Occasionally, a relative or an acquaintance would travel and bring news.

The following chapters will expand upon most of these stories. There were several nodal points that highlight the narrative. For instance, the sudden illness and death of Benjamin Cohen. One day during 1934, his health began to deteriorate with no apparent reason. Help was sought amongst local doctors in Salonica but to no avail. No fruitful diagnosis could be reached. As a last resort, the family raised enough resources and sought consultation with a renowned consultant in Vienna. The diagnosis was grim. Several months later, Benjamin was dead. All the while, his illness and death were kept a secret from his sister Rita in Palestine. She was pregnant with her third child, and the family believed that the news of her beloved young brother's illness and death would adversely affect her pregnancy.

It was hard to keep up the cover-up for very long. Rita sensed something was wrong and kept pestering her mother, sister and brothers for news. She asked for photographs to be sent, as was customary in those days, and as these were not forthcoming, her suspicion rose higher and higher. It was only six months after his death that she was told. And even then, it was not done directly. First her husband, Shmuel, was told and asked to keep it to himself. In fact, it was Benjamin who introduced his good friend Shmuel Parenti to his sister Rita. At the same time of Benjamin's illness and towards his death, Leon's wife was also entering the last phase of her first pregnancy in Paris. When he was born in 1935, the baby was named Benjamin.

During 1936, much focus was placed upon the hardship that Rita and Shmuel endured in Palestine. Already the parents of three young children, the couple struggled to support the growing family's needs.

Shmuel was trying to provide for the family by selling merchandise on the streets of Tel Aviv and Jaffa. The family lived in poverty but still fared better than the family they left behind in Salonica. Occasionally, they were able to send money, small gifts and medical requirements. It was during 1936 that the news of the Arab uprising against the small Jewish community, and against the British rule in Palestine, filled many pages of correspondence.

After Benjamin's untimely death, probably due to insufficient medical treatment caused by the poverty and the harsh conditions in Salonica in those days, came the prospects of Sami's wedding. Sami's wedding was supposed to be an occasion for celebration in August 1937. He asked and received from his older bachelor brothers, Dino and Eli, permission to wed before they did. Such was the custom. The bride to be was from a good local Jewish family. All seemed well. The family was looking forward to the happy event, and it was written about in abundance. But then, an inspection in the office where Sami worked revealed that there were too many clerks working there, and as he was the last to be engaged in employment, he lost his post. Upon hearing that the groom had lost his job and the only source of income, the bride's family cancelled the wedding promptly, causing much pain to the Cohens, locally and abroad.

And then, in November 1938, Rachelle Cohen, the mother of the family, became sick with the flu and within days contracted angina and, despite medical efforts, died. The shock was immense. A string of dark and sad letters were sent to Paris and Palestine. Letters of condolences and sorrow. For Rita in Palestine and Leon and Isaac in Paris, these news were even harder. They last saw their mother five or more years previously. They could not properly part from her. They were cut off from their homeland and now also from their mother, this time for good.

The year 1939 brought with it the prospects of war. The German army is in Paris. Fear and dread are strewn in the letters exchanged between Paris, Palestine and Salonica. Everyone was struggling with economic difficulties and now also burdened with worsening political times. The family's backbone is now Ines. Despite her personal financial hardship and deteriorating dental health, she continued to write letters and to reproach her brothers for not doing more. She struggled to maintain some sort of family life for the extended family as well as her own. Her relationship with her sister Rita in Palestine was very important for her. She understood how much Rita missed her home and made a special effort to keep her informed, though there were very few happy items of news to communicate.

The letters become scarcer and scarcer during 1940 and the beginning of 1941. In 1941, the Germans are already in Salonica and the worst is beginning to take place. The very last letter that was sent from Salonica to Palestine is dated February 1st 1941. Its content is not very different from others. It ends though with the ominous sentence written by Ines: *"We are still hoping and waiting for better days"*. That was the last recorded communication from the Cohen family in Salonica.

As described earlier, the letters were discovered gradually over a period of more than ten years. From the beginning, they evoked a mix of reactions from Rita's five children.

One brother showed some scepticism and thought the process of delving into the letters was futile. As far as he was concerned, the only worthwhile outcome of dealing with the letters and the clues they provided would be if they led to the discovery of some lost relatives. He had hoped that two of Rita's brothers, Sam and Dino, who might have joined the partisans, managed to survive the war, settled somewhere and raised families. He had hoped that it would be possible to trace them. It did not take long before it became clear that such efforts would lead nowhere, and soon, he lost interest in the pursuit of the lost relatives in particular and in the letters in general. Still, he remained curious and supportive of the efforts of the other siblings.

A different reaction altogether was found in a younger brother. He took it upon himself to collate, translate and bring to print all the found letters of the first and second boxes. This he did with the help and co-operation of his oldest sister. It was in fact a mutual project in which he was the executing force while she supported it. The work on the letters deepened the already deep relationship between them.

The other two sisters reacted each in their own way. They both felt a deep sense of obligation to preserve the testimony of the letters but with a varying sense of commitment. They both showed interest and involvement but with less actual contribution to the work involved. This had soon become a source of tension, erupting often in acrimonious accusations, leading to long periods of angry silences and alternating with weak and half-hearted attempts at reconciliation.

Endless anecdotes could be told about the various twists in this sad tale of anger, break-up, reconciliation and hurt pride since the parents had died in relative old age and the letters were discovered. The pertinent question in my view is whether those complex, but not out-of-the-ordinary familial difficulties, can be understood in the particular life circumstances that the family developed, in particular in the light of the traumatic response the mother of the family had towards the loss of all her family in the Holocaust.

In order to explain my claim, it is necessary to recount briefly the history of the family's arrival in Palestine in the 1930s. Rita was the second daughter of the Cohen family who lived in Salonica. As already mentioned, she married Shmuel Parenti who was younger than her. He devoted his time to various Zionist activities in Salonica. It was clear to him that, once married, he would emigrate to Palestine and so serve as an example to the rest of the Jewish community. Indeed, in 1930, he married Rita, and two years later, she gave birth to the first child, Esther.

A few months later, as soon as the young mother and her baby were able to travel, they found themselves on the boat to Palestine. The rest of Rita's family stayed behind, not being as Zionist-inclined as Shmuel. Like many Jews at that time, they viewed the growing Jewish settlement of Palestine with sympathy and support but did not feel compelled to leave their country behind. One can understand that without a zeal for the move or extreme necessity, most people would prefer to stay within their familiar surroundings and hope that present conditions would improve and allow them to continue as before. A few, like Shmuel, were gripped both by the Zionist mission as well as having within them the nomadic personality that enabled them to take the risk, uproot themselves and seek new horizons.

The new family began its life in Palestine. The conditions were tough. Poverty was common, and it was hard for Shmuel to provide for his new family. Soon, more births followed – first another girl, Zmira, then a boy child Shlomo and finally, the twins Benjamin and Rachel (both named after Rita's dead brother and mother).

During all that time, the situation in Europe worsened. As the letters testify, the Cohens who stayed in Europe, like the rest of the Jews, faced greater and greater persecution, worsened by the bleak prospects that the Nazi regime offered in the future.

In 1939, in Palestine, Rita was receiving worrying news. She tried to concentrate on the present time, being a mother of five young children, having to cope with tough physical and economic conditions, surrounded by a political climate where the future of the new state-to-be was often threatened the hostility of the Arab countries surrounding it. To make things worse, her health was deteriorating. Four successful births, and quite a few miscarriages, made things tougher and tougher, and she had no choice but to lean more and more on the help of her eldest daughter who was even required to quit her schooling at the age of 12 in order to earn money to support the family economy as well as shoulder some of the house chores.

Rita's heart was torn. The demands of daily life required her full attention, but her heart was elsewhere, with her brothers, sister and mother in Salonica. Like many of her contemporaries who had arrived in Palestine, she tried to be a part of the new world but could not deny to herself the links to the old one.

She waited for the letters daily. Their arrival was both a respite from the daily chores as well as a point of great sorrow. She could follow her family through the letters and feel a part of the home she left behind. On the other hand, she felt increasingly helpless in regard to their hardships. She was aware that they were not telling her all. Some news came muted, dispersed and coded. She had to read between the lines, to guess, to piece together. She could tell that things were not going well all the time.

She shared these experiences with her immediate neighbours, many of whom, in the poor shabby neighbourhood she lived, were in similar situations. They too received letters. They too found themselves torn between the two worlds.

Her growing children, on the other hand, showed little interest. She could understand that. They were children, making their first steps into the world. Their lives were exciting. Living in the new land was all they ever knew about. They had nowhere else they could think of. They had nowhere else they could feel torn from, longing for. They were content with their lives, however humble they were in material terms.

Whenever she tried to tell them about her family back in Salonica, they listened, or seemed to listen, looked briefly at the photos she showed them and turned away as soon as possible, perhaps unconsciously trying to defend themselves from what felt like overwhelming grief.

Turning to her husband was not much help either. He was busy making the ends meet. He was a kind man, and she could rely on him in many aspects of their mutual lives. But his circumstances were different from hers in at least one significant aspect. He managed to bring his immediate nuclear family with him. Both his parents and sister emigrated to Palestine soon after him and settled nearby, even though he too was saddened by the loss of his uncles who had stayed behind.[49] They were a source of support for him, but for her, they were a grievance. His mother never really liked her for reasons she could never fathom. Was it because she was relatively old when they married? Was it because of the rumours surrounding her previous relationships with men in Salonica before she married Shmuel? Was it the legendary common dislike mothers-in-law have towards their sons' wives? Regardless of the reason, she felt estranged from her and knew that her husband favoured his mother enough for her not to put his loyalty to the test.

She remained mostly within herself regarding the emotional impact the letters had upon her. That withdrawal had a price. It is possible to say that Rita suffered a chronic depressive reaction following those years of uncertainty, which were followed by even worse news when the reality of the Holocaust became known.

This of course was a gradual process. First, news of Jews being deported, rounded up and sent to camps arrived. Then, the worse news of the concentration camps and the gas chambers. Those news filtered in even during the war years themselves but reverberated much more strongly after the war ended and the first survivors began arriving in Palestine.

Rita was a mother of five children in 1945, when the war ended. Her eldest was thirteen and her two young twins were six. She was devastated. Though hopes that some of her brothers and sister and their siblings somehow survived the war persisted for years, she knew that that was not true. She felt that they were dead. She began the long process of mourning that never ended, not until she herself was dead, forty years later in 1986.[50]

Rita's deep mourning affected not only her. As she was also physically not well, she needed her eldest daughter to share more and more of the housekeeping duties and mothering responsibilities with her. Esther had no choice but to do what was required of her. She became the second mother for her siblings and especially the young twins. She was given certain authorities in the house and carried them out as well as she could and to the best of her thirteen-year-old sensibilities. She was made to quit school. She had to go to work to earn more money for the household. In between, she tried to stay loyal to her enthusiastic devotion to her youth movement activities. But one could say that her childhood days ended sooner than anticipated.

Coupled with the discriminatory paternal regime that meant that boys were more important than girls, this change of maternal care had an insidious and lasting effect upon the relationships between the siblings. It is during these years that the seeds of later eruptions were sown.

The creation of the uncanny

The family was held together by necessity during the 1940s and the years that followed. Israel was recognized as an independent state in 1948 by the UN, which perhaps gave Rita a sense of pride and purpose, but did not alleviate the grave sense of loss. On the contrary, during the early days of the state, it was difficult to give full weight to the emotional, mental and physical pain and suffering that emanated from the loss of the European Jewry. It was almost commonly held that in order for the young, at-war state to survive and thrive, it was necessary to shed the links to the past, including references to the Holocaust.

It was not that the Holocaust was denied on a conscious level immediately after the end of the war. In some aspects, such as receiving vast amounts of compensation money from post-war West Germany during the 1950s, it was even used as a lever against the international community to favour the Zionist interest at the expense of the significant Arab population in Israel. But its true impact was delegated to the nether realms of the collective soul. It was a time for daily struggle with the many challenges of living in a state surrounded by Arab enemies who threatened its very existence. It was not yet time to look back into the catastrophe that the Jewish people suffered in Europe.

All of her children went on to marry, raise children and lead good professional lives during the 1960s and 1970s. In her little flat, both she and her husband welcomed the growing family on Friday afternoon for black coffee and Borakeetas.[51] It always seemed like a beehive of merriment. The grandchildren running around in the little flat, the grown-ups sitting around and exchanging tales of that week's happenings, one big happy family.

Rita would sit on her green armchair, always slightly leaning forward as if wanting to be more involved, listening intently, her maternal regality permeating the situation. Each grandchild would have his or her moment of glory on her knees. She always showed keen interest in them. She told each of her own children how wonderful their children were. She showed great pride. Her light green eyes would easily water with excitement as she watched them, as she patted their hair and pulled them towards her for a big crushing loving hug. She would hug them till they squealed with joy mixed with pain.

The nodal point of her contact with her grandchildren, especially the older ones, which sometimes happened immediately as they entered the flat, at other times later, but always there as a reminder, would be the moment she would pull out the large photo album that was on the coffee table, always there. It was a photo album with heavy wooden covers and brass engravings upon it, depicting the Western Wall in Jerusalem. She would open and turn the pages. They would then look at the black and white photos of her deceased siblings. The photos were faded mostly, small in size. She would point to each of them in turn, say their name and after each name fix her gaze upon the grandchild. She would then compare the dead sibling to one of her children and, in later years, to one of her grandchildren. She would extoll some virtue she remembered and find clues to them in the behaviour or achievement of one of the children or grandchildren in the room.

It seemed that each dead sibling, or their off-spring, had a live extension in the room, a breathing monument, *a doppelgänger*. She would utter their name, trembling, already tears welling up in her green eyes, point to the photo and then point to the grandchild present. It was an uncanny moment. As if she was transforming the dead into the living. As if she was transferring their souls, their memories, with the movement of her index finger and the firm green gaze of her eyes.

Whoever stood in front of her felt this to be a sacred moment. It was as if she was giving the child his life as well as the dead siblings' life. "Remember them", she would plead and command at the same time. She would then wipe her tears, deride herself in some way and try to move on as quickly as possible. The moment was brief, lasting not more than a minute or so at the most. And yet, it seemed to me to be the highlight and most poignant moment throughout the whole afternoon.

Often, the others present in the room would not notice it, and if they did, they did not intervene. That small ritual had to be performed and not be interrupted. If the grandchild was upset in some way by her emotion, they would be gathered into their parents' arms, cooed briefly and then go back to play with the others.

Quite often, being the eldest of her grandchildren, it was I who was sat on her lap, it was I who was entrusted with this painful memory, it was I who was given the memory to hold, the gaze to contain, the tears that would wash over into my soft and impressionable soul.

The evolution of my postmemory – psychoanalytic considerations

For most of my life, I carried the memory of Leon Cohen within me as a cherished object. Intuitively, I felt that I was given a rare gift. I felt that Rita entrusted me with a part of her being. It made me feel special. It made me feel proud. I felt that I was chosen by her to carry something. As a child, I did not comprehend what it was I was meant to carry but I knew that it was mine to hold and cherish. I did not think much about it. It just was part of me.

But that gift turned out to be a live object, my postmemory, as I began to understand in later years. It had many uncanny appearances in my life, three of which I will now recount.

The first one was upon her death in 1986. I was living in England at the time and received the news two weeks later through a letter. I was told that in her purse was only one item – a letter which I had written to her several weeks before. That letter was read aloud at the funeral. I felt that familiar mixed emotion – on the one hand, I grieved her loss and, in addition, felt anger that I was not notified in time, and on the other hand, I experienced the narcissistic joy of being unique, being the chosen one. It was *my* letter that she had kept in her otherwise empty purse. It felt again as if I had a special role in her life, one which I kept hoping I was fulfilling. I could not yet say what it was exactly but felt driven to stay attentive to a voice that I believed was speaking to me.

The second one came a few years later while I was studying for my B.A. degree in Photography. I had to write a thesis, and when thinking of a possible subject, I decided that I would write about photographs relating to the Holocaust, initially not knowing exactly what particular angle I would choose to explore. Again, it felt like I responded to some inner calling that set me on a course without being consciously aware of the origin of the call. As I progressed in the research, I focused upon the notion of *the concerned photographer* and in particular the figure of Roman Vishniac (1897–1990) who was a Jewish Russian photographer who sensed that the tide was changing for European Jewry and began a huge project of documenting the lives of various communities in Eastern Europe.[52] He survived the war but stopped taking photographs of people, which I claimed was his traumatized reaction to the Holocaust. When asking myself as to why I decided upon this topic, which was at the time not in line with my other cultural and artistic preoccupations, all I could think of was Rita's figure. My intuition was that I owed it to her.

When trying to understand what it was that I owed her, I came against a blank. I did not know. I just knew that I owed it to her to do this work on the Holocaust in memory of her brothers. I dedicated the thesis to her and added an inscription from Pirkei Avot 2:16 – "You are not obligated to complete the work, but neither are you free to desist from it". That too was an uncharacteristic choice for me as I was totally unfamiliar with Pirkei Avot but came across that sentence accidently.

The third took place years later when I was back in Israel, during the first decade of this century. Again, as with the two previous ones, it had to do with my writing. When I decided to write a Ph.D. thesis, I knew almost immediately that I would write it on the subject of writers who have spent a significant time of their lives away from their homeland, in exile. I knew I wanted to explore the idea that one could write best on his connection with home, only once he was removed from it by necessity or by choice. The idea echoes many psychoanalytic notions regarding attachment and independence. It felt to be the work of my life.

After much deliberation, I decided to focus upon the work of Lawrence Durrell's (1912–1990) *The Alexandria Quartet,* which he wrote in between 1958 and 1960. The tetralogy tells the story of a young English teacher who arrived in Alexandria just before the outbreak of World War II. He falls in love with a local beauty, Justine. Each of the four volumes of the tetralogy tells the narrative from a different perspective, thus creating a labyrinthine tale where it is hard to pinpoint the truth. I used psychoanalytic ideas to study the work, focusing on themes like dreams, fiction versus reality, exile and homeland and more.

I finished the work and was awarded with the degree in 2013 and since then also had it published both in Hebrew and English.[53] But when asked why I specifically chose to write about, I never felt fully satisfied with the answers I gave and deep down could not really say why I chose that particular work after all.

It was only during one of my therapy sessions that I came to a deeper understanding of my unconscious motivation. Going back in my mind to Rita's lap as she showed me the photos of her siblings, pointing to each one in turn, saying their name and then looking at me to make sure I understood.

The one name that she repeated more than others was the name of her younger brother Leon. Why she chose to single him out to me will never be known. Perhaps, there **was** some physical resemblance, as I was told in later years. While telling all this to my therapist, it suddenly dawned on me that both Leon Cohen and Lawrence Durrell were living at Paris during the same very years, the 1930s. The emotional reaction I experienced when realising the connection indicated that it was not likely to just be a coincidence. Could it be that my *conscious* choice of Lawrence Durrell as a subject was a result of an *unconscious* infantile confusion that riveted on that biographical detail, insignificant in itself? Could it be that I had internalised the fact the detail about Leon's stay in Paris during the 1930s and confused it with Durrell's sojourn there? Could it be that my research of Durrell's life was in effect *a displaced* research into Leon's life? Could it be that I was unconsciously *compelled to repeat* an infantile memory so as to try answer my grandmother's wish to find her dead brother? Was *the finding* of Lawrence Durrell an unconscious *wish fulfilment* of that *primal scene* whereby I was given my life's mission by my grandmother *to remember* her dead siblings?

To try and understand the evolution of my postmemory, I refer to two of Freud's concepts. It is not by accident that it is Freud, of all possible theoreticians, that I chose. Being one of the most influential intellectuals of the twentieth century, he also lived in Europe during some of the same period. As is known, he was able to flee Vienna in 1938 with the aid of his disciple, the princess Marie Bonaparte (1882–1962). He managed to save his wife and children but had to leave behind his sisters who were killed in the concentration camps. Incidentally, I found out when I visited the street in Paris where Leon and his family lived before taken away by the French police in November 1942, Rue le Goff near Jardin de Luxembourg, that Freud stayed in the hotel opposite the Cohens in 1885 during his three-month fellowship, when he studied with Jean-Martin Charcot (1825–1893), a renowned neurologist who was conducting scientific research into hypnosis. In the later years, he described that period as catalytic in showing him the way towards the practice of medical psychopathology and then psychoanalysis. It is perhaps incidental and arbitrary, and yet, I have come to think of those terms in a different light.

The two Freudian concepts I use are *screen memory* (1899) and *the uncanny* (1919). Freud's paper *screen memory* is an early paper that was written at the same time he was working on his seminal work on dreams (1900). In this paper, Freud describes a common clinical phenomenon whereby a patient would present a vivid, almost unreal and persistent childhood memory that seems in itself significant but is not so significant as to explain its persistence and its vivid and yet unreal clarity. The memory itself remains unaltered through the patient's life. Freud claimed that the *screen memory* points out to a deeper, more objectionable, repressed memory.[54]

The memory I retained of myself as a child sitting on Rita's lap and following her fingers as she pointed out one brother after the other, calling them by names and describing their characteristics and then pointing out to us and making analogies, is such a *screen memory*.

The repressed content that was hidden from my consciousness was the association Rita made between me and her brother Leon. As a child, it was not possible for me to contain the association. Being given such a heritage was a burden I had to repress. What I could not keep conscious was my ambivalent reaction towards my beloved grandmother at such a gift. It felt like an act of aggression. Why would my beloved grandmother want to give me such a toxic present? It was one thing to be considered her chosen grandson but quite another to become a living memorial for a dead brother, murdered in the Holocaust. Through the process of splitting, I was able to repress the aggressive aspects of that gift that implant and only preserve consciously the positive and loving aspects of the bond that she formed with me by associating me with her brother.

The repressed element of the split remained buried deeply, occasionally sending up signals like the urge to write about the Holocaust. It also created symptoms such as an almost compulsive attraction to materials regarding the Holocaust and a tendency to cry easily and with no clear reason at certain times and event associated with the tragic loss of children and relatives.

Freud's *the uncanny* helps to illustrate how that repressed element worked underground all these years until it did find a creative and relatively healthy form of expression through the writing of my doctoral thesis.[55]

What Freud meant by *the uncanny* is quite complex. Using several literary figures, Freud claimed that the common phenomenon whereby we think that something familiar is in fact foreign to us or vice versa is based on a developmental process that takes place early in childhood. Freud writes that what we do as children in order to accommodate new sensual, emotional and cognitive experience in early childhood is to create a duplicate image of ourselves that accommodates the new data as a transitory receptacle until it is fully absorbed into our growing and developing sense of self. In later years, as the emotional and cognitive apparatus matures, the duplicate mechanism becomes redundant and obsolete and sinks into oblivion. But it never completely disappears. Occasionally, and according to Freud at times of emotional stress, the mental apparatus is reactivated, and we experience familiar and immediate reality as if it is new and foreign to us, and conversely, unfamiliar sensual information echoes a familiarity within us that is inexplicable through logical thinking.

Leon Cohen's memory and the associated emotional significance that I sensed was applied to it by my grandmother was subjected to the uncanny process. My choice of Lawrence Durrell as the subject for my thesis, which I had thought of and spoken of as the work of my life, originated from the ambivalent identification with the memory and the emotional imperative associated with Leon Cohen, based upon the seemingly trivial biographical detail that they both shared – living in Paris in the 1930s.

By exploring the work and life of Lawrence Durrell, I was in fact unconsciously trying to retrace the whereabouts of Leon Cohen in that same city at that time, just before he was captured with his wife and two children by the Nazis. What I was perhaps mostly writing about was the city itself, Paris, Salonica, Tel Aviv, any city that served as the liminal stage for the individual in his quest for meaning.

Leon Cohen was the hidden uncanny figure of my thesis that explored the connection the individual has to his real and fictitious homeland. A connection that can best be explored through writing.

In his 1908 essay *Creative Writing and Day-dreaming*, Freud tries to outline what it is that motivates the individual to write creatively to explore his psyche through the act of writing.[56] What does such an individual possess, or what possesses him, to enable him to engage in the creative process, deemed by Western culture as the ultimate form of individual achievement?

Freud asks whether we should not look for the first traces of imaginative activity as early as in childhood? The child's best-loved and most intense occupation is with his play or games. Might we not say that every child at play behaves like a creative writer, in that he creates a world of his own, or, rather, re-arranges the things in his world in a new way that pleases him?

So, if the origins of the creative act, and the depth of the wound, are to be discovered and traced back to childhood, it is only natural that we should follow Freud's suggestion and seek answers and insights regarding the interpretation of the appearance of my postmemory in that early memory.

I believe that it was my interest in the letters as a way of trying to bring back to life the Cohen family that led me to almost accidentally write my doctoral thesis. Once I had realized that, having completed the thesis and got it published, I was left with a sense that the mission was not yet completed. The imperative I was given was not quite fulfilled. And perhaps it can never be fully fulfilled, such is the nature of trauma. The following chapters, each dedicated to one of the twenty years between 1923 and 1942, is my *postmemorial* work. In each of the chapters, I quote the majority of the letters from that year, as well as adding further information, so as to allow the reader into the real, and imagined, lives of the Cohens. Each of the chapters can be read as a standalone testimony, while the flow of the years altogether allows a deeper perspective of those fatal years in Europe, not only to the Cohens from Salonica, but to humanity itself.

Notes

1 There is more research on the fate of the Jews in France during World War II than in Greece. For further reading regarding the fate of the Jews in France, read Cohen's 1996, *The Shoah in France* and Saul Friedländer's 1978 *When Memory Comes*. Friedländer though born in Prague survived the war in France as he was hidden in a Catholic school. It is harder to find comprehensive reading on the fate of the Jews in Greece, but a good recent starting point is Moses' and Antoniou's 2018 book, *The Holocaust in Greece*. To the best of my knowledge, there is no specific research published upon the story of Greek Jews who had emigrated to France before World War II and who were deported to the concentration camps.

2 Hoffman, 1990.

3 As early as 1896, in his *Further Remarks on the Neuro-Psychoses of Defence*, Sigmund Freud (1856–1939) referred to the idea of the *return of the repressed*,

i.e. emergence of unconscious material that had been repressed as a result of representing ideas and sensations which the ego could not tolerate at the time of their occurrence, either due to the immaturity of the individual or due to their severance and threat. As this is not a purely psychoanalytic essay, I refer for further reading on this, and other Freudian terms, to Laplance's and Pontalis' excellent 1973 book, *The Language of Psychoanalysis.*

4 The concept of postmemory was conceived by several thinkers over the last few decades. I refer to its interpretation as explained by Hoffman and Frosh.

5 I have chosen to use throughout the book the old variant Salonica as the name of the city rather than the original Thessaloniki, named after Alexander the Great's half-sister, the Macedonian princess, Thessalonike of Macedon, 345 BCE. Salonica was the name the city was known by throughout the world since the twelfth century. In 1912, after the Greek state regained control of the city, the original name was reinstated. However, throughout the letters and in the family memory, the name Salonica was used, probably because of its usage in Ladino. In some of the letters, the Cohens warn that they now must use the official name Thessaloniki so as to avoid reprisals such as seizure of letters.

6 Wiesel, 1958.

7 The scope of this book, or its aim, is not sufficient to explore in-depth further details of the history of Salonica beyond aspects which are pertinent to this particular story. For further reading about the history of the Jewish community of Salonica, one usually begins with Mazower's 2005 book on Salonica and Keridis' and Kiesling's 2020 book on Thessaloniki. Mazower's book's publication and its translation into many languages have changed the historiography of the city, bringing to light not only the rich texture of what was thought of as *the madre de Israel* but also more controversial and violent events in the city's history. Another good source is volume 28 of *The Jewish History*, a special issue dedicated to Salonica's Jews, which brings together essays by a group of scholars who have brought together many unique perspectives to try and present different views of the Jewish community of Salonica than the traditional view which had represented the community as a homogenous entity, disregarding many significant complex issues. Following the publication of Mazower's book, a yearly seminar was held in Salonica for seven years, led by Yorgos Antoniou, Henriette Benveniste, Paris Papamichos Chronakis and Anthony Molho. In 2014, another international conference was held at the International Hellenic University in Salonica, Holocaust in Greece: Genocide and its Aftermath. I had the privilege of being invited to present the early stages of my research during that conference. For a native Greek account of the expulsion of the Jews from Salonica, read Yorgos Ioannou's *And it came to pass ...* in his 1997 collection of prose and essays about the city, *Refugee Capital.* For a plausible fictional description of the city, read Victoria Hislop's *The Thread.*

8 Salonica's 500 years' old Jewish Cemetery was expropriated and desecrated on December 1942 by the local municipalities, and about 100,000 graves were robbed of their valuable marble gravestones and sold to local churches and contractors who used the marble as building materials throughout the city. It was only in 2014 that the local municipality acknowledged its part in this atrocity and erected a small monument on a very small section of the site of the cemetery, which has been used after the end of the war to build the Aristotle University on the burial grounds. The monument has since been desecrated several times by local Neo-Nazis groups. For further reading on the history of the cemetery, read Devin E. Naar's 2016 book, *Jewish Salonica.*

9 Saltiel's recent well-researched 2020 book, *The Holocaust in Thessaloniki*, details the way local Christian and Municipal institutions in Salonica aide the Nazis in the destruction of the Jewish community.

10 As described at length in a 2017 book edited by Zalc and Bruttmann, *Microhistory* refers to research concerning particular case studies of individuals, families and communities.

11 Felman, 2000.

12 Frosh, 2019.

13 Yad Vashem (Hebrew: יד ושם; literally, "a monument and a name") is Israel's official memorial to the victims of the Holocaust. It is dedicated to preserving the memory of the dead; honouring Jews who fought against their Nazi oppressors and non-Jews who selflessly aided Jews in need; and researching the phenomenon of the Holocaust in particular and genocide in general, with the aim of avoiding such events in the future.

14 It is also possible, of course, that Isaac had already left Salonica when the picture was taken, but that the grimace on Leon's face suggests that he was intimate with the person taking the photograph. This, like many other questions, will remain unresolved.

15 The Bourla family was a well-to-do family of bankers and merchants. Alas, my branch of the family did not enjoy any privileges. Furthermore, it appears that in times of need, and there were many, the few attempts to gain help from the Bourla side of the family met with stringent and cold refusals.

16 The given names of the Parenti children were originally Sephardic, but as was, unfortunately, the custom in the burgeoning Jewish community in Palestine in the 1930s, they were switched to more "proper" Hebrew sounding names. Thus, Nina became Esther, Martha became Zmira, etc., the attachment to the original names remained, and in their eighties, they referred back to their original names. This was quite a common phenomenon in the early days of Israel, and most Jewish immigrant communities underwent some process of adaptation and shedding off their original tradition (often referred to as *the melting pot*). During the 1990s, an ever-growing trend in Israeli society celebrates the original cultures left behind, including reclaiming names and the growth in the use and study of the local Jewish dialects, such as Ladino. Ladino was the mother tongue of the Cohens. Even after emigrating to Israel, it was the language spoken in Rita's household, and all of Rita's children speak it fluently to this day. Unfortunately, it was not passed down to my generation, and thus, we have suffered the loss of this beautiful, poetic and proverbial tongue.

   The scope of this book cannot do justice to any of that, beyond this endnote.

17 As is described in the chapter on 1942, two references to a Samuel Cohen from Salonica were found during the research for this book. Neither was confirmed as Rita's and Leon's brother.

18 For further reading, see Alfandary, 2020.

19 For further reading, see Fleming's 2014 article, "Salonica's Jews".

20 A cursive form of the Hebrew alphabet, traditionally, a Sephardi script, Solitreo is nonetheless the predecessor of the modern Ashkenazi Cursive Hebrew currently used for handwriting in modern Israel and for Yiddish. In Judaeo-Spanish ("Ladino") of the Balkans and Turkey, it served as the standard handwritten form that complemented the Rashi script character set used for printing.

21 Saltiel, 2017.

22 Ginio, 2002.

23 Rafael, 2001.

24 Various people took part in the translations of the letters: the letters in the first
    two boxes were translated by Moshe Bacher, Rachel Wolf, Avner Peretz, Helen
    Lotan and Eliezer Papo. The Solitreo letters were translated by Dr. Dov Haco-
    hen. The letters from the third box were translated by Lizette Leichner, and the
    letters from the fourth box were translated by Dr. Emanuel Cohen and Mari-
    anne Leloir.
25 Derrida, 1960.
26 Freud, 1919.
27 A small neighbourhood where around eighty people lived during the mid-1930s,
    on the banks of the Ayalon (Wadi Musrara). The neighbourhood was adjacent
    to Sova Bakery (nowadays, the route of the tunnel that descends from La Guar-
    dia Junction to South Ayalon Highway).
28 At first, she even denied having ever known Isaac or Rita. This is contradicted
    by some letters where Isaac writes that he is trying to find a match for her. One
    very clear evidence of the very close ties Rosette had with Leon and Bondy is
    the fact that the collection contains dozens of picture postcards she sent to the
    couple in their Rue le Goff address.
29 The letters in the first and second boxes were translated and lovingly compiled
    into a printed booklet by the younger brother Benjamin Parenti (Parran) with
    the help of his brother and sisters and their spouses. That booklet is a family
    treasure as it also contains statements by the siblings.
30 Zweig, 1938.
31 Collingwood, 1993.
32 Montaigne, 2004.
33 Comments written in the letters by Rony Alfandary will appear in brackets and
    in regular type.
34 One of the signatories on that appointment letter was Shlomo Nehama, a rel-
    ative of Joseph Nehama who wrote the definitive, seven-volume Histoire des
    Israélites de Salonique published in 1935.
35 For a thorough survey of the various political groups in the Jewish community
    of Salonica in the inter-war years can be found in Naar's 2016 book. For further
    details about the life in the Hirsch Quarter and the deportation of the Jews from
    it, read Matarasso's 2020 book.
36 For further reading, refer to Aymard's 2014 article.
37 One of the outcomes of the dominance of the Alliance Israélite Universelle in
    the educational scene of Salonican Jews was a cultural affinity to life in France.
    Apart from the obvious advantage of being fluent in French, it was a country
    many middle-class, educated Salonica Jews aspired to live in, not unlike the
    draw Zionist Jews had towards emigrating to Palestine.
38 The list is available online https://www.ushmm.org/.
39 Levi, 1979.
40 Founded in Paris in 1860 by a group of emancipated French Jews, the Alliance
    Israélite Universelle's goal was to "offer effective support to those who suffer for
    being Jewish". In order to achieve its aim of "working everywhere towards the
    emancipation and progress of Jews", the Alliance concentrated on the creation
    of a vast educational network in the Balkans, the Near and Middle East and
    in North Africa. The Salonica branch opened in 1874. The Alliance was not
    a pro-Zionist organization and saw its aim to integrate the Jewish communi-
    ties in their European countries. Rita's association with the Alliance, therefore,
    throws further light upon her reluctance to emigrate to Palestine with her Zion-
    ist husband. For further reading, refer to Molho's 1993 article "Education in the
    Jewish Community of Thessaloniki in the Beginning of the 20th Century".

41 In his 1997 novel, Gioconda, the Greek author Níkos Kokántzis wrote about an illicit love affair between a Jewish Salonica woman and a Greek man in the years before World War II. In the novel, their love affair is brought to a tragic stop when he was not able to save her from being sent by the Nazis and the local police to her death in Auschwitz. Would that have been Rita's fate if she was allowed to continue her relationship with her Christian lover?

42 Theodore Herzl Association and Degel Sion (mentioned later) were Salonica-based Zionist organizations. More information about them can be found in The Central Archives for the History of the Jewish People in Jerusalem (CAHJP).

43 Reik, 1948.

44 Joffo, 2001.

44 Reik, 1948.

46 Bachelard, 1994.

47 Winnicott, 1960.

48 The scope and intention of this book do not allow for further detailed analysis of the subjects of local collaboration with the Nazis and the struggles that took place around the formation of Israel. For French collaboration, read Joly's 2018 and Saltiel's 2020 books. Regarding the formation of Israel, a good place to start might be Segev's 2013 book.

49 Most of his uncles and their families had remained in Salonica and perished in the Holocaust. The few that survived were suspected of being collaborators. The scope of this study does not allow more details on this subject.

50 During the early 1950s, she and Shmuel registered their dead relatives in Daf-Ed, Yad Vashem's project of registering the victims of the Holocaust.

51 Small cheese pastries.

52 In 2016, an article I wrote about Vishniac and *the concerned photographer* was published in Hebrew in the Alaxon on-line magazine. A later version was also included in a book published in 2020, also in Hebrew.

53 Alfandary, 2019.

54 Freud, 1899.

55 Freud, 1919.

56 Freud, 1908.

Part II

The letters

1923 – Beginnings

Leon Cohen (1901–1942). He only lived until he was forty-one. Of that I can be sure though I was not there when he died. As I am writing this, right now, I have lived almost twenty years longer than he had. Yet, despite that, I am ready to tell his/my story (Figure 14).

For me, Leon Cohen is not even a personal memory. And yet, he is perhaps the person who has influenced me the most, unknowingly. It has taken me the best part of fifty years to realise. Will I have enough time left to fully come to terms with what his memory has left behind in my mind?

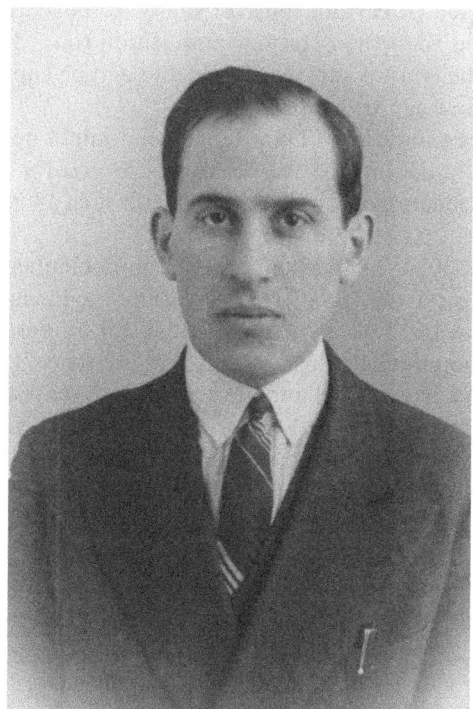

Figure 14 Leon Cohen.

I was born in 1962, twenty years after he and his family were murdered in Auschwitz. When I write that he is not a personal memory, I am stating the obvious. How can I remember someone who died twenty years before I was even born? And yet, I insist that his presence has been haunting me from as early as I can remember myself. As remote as his presence seems to be from me at my present moment, it is a distance I know I can travel through reading the letters in his collection so as to increase the intimacy I feel towards his memory. Reaching an intimacy with anyone requires first to acknowledge the distance in between. The distance will be overcome, gradually, word by word, as I make his presence un-transparent, as I recognize his distinctiveness, his connectiveness. It is a journey I must make within myself in order to reach that deeply buried memory, so as to transform my postmemory into a living and intimate presence.

When writing a history, be it a history of so few details, the dominant forces in the text are the questions asked about the missing details. The forming of the question is in itself a complex process. There is an argument concerning the nature and depth of questioning desired or allowed in certain situations. The depth and sharpness of the questions are tightly linked to what is desired as knowledge. Some knowledge can be threatening, and therefore, we allow it to remain undisturbed under layers of not knowing and not questioning. Issues of shame and privacy create a filter in the mind of the researcher, guiding him towards safer grounds. Family taboos may need to be protected. A certain sense of safety in the world may appear to be more important than the persistent inquisition towards truth, knowing in advance that the truth is forever elusive and can be captured only to the extent that a shadow can be captured.

Dare I ask all the questions? Dare I face what might be revealed? I want to see what's really behind that terrible tag – *Holocaust Victim*. I am not satisfied with the generalizations associated with such an identity in this age of Identity Politics.

George Steiner (1929–2020) asked an even more eloquent question in his autobiographical study *Errata* in 1997 regarding the formation of memory. He asked how can the senses, through the brain, impose a coherent and clear narrative upon the kaleidoscopic vista of existence.[1]

Steiner's father was watchful and alert enough to sense the danger in Europe and in December 1942, only a month after the Nazi forces occupied Paris, took his family and moved to the USA, where Steiner pursued a career as a world-renowned scholar. Being Viennese Jews by origin, that move was the second, and the final, that the family had made in those years. His father, Frederick George, had read the signs well and, in 1924, took his family away from their native city of Vienna to Paris, where young George was born. He invested in the linguistic education of his children and equipped them with a fluency in what Steiner thought of as his three mother tongues: German, English and French. It was that second move from Paris to the USA that saved their lives.

Leon Cohen, like many Salonica Jews of his generation, was fluent in French and Ladino, with some command of Greek and Turkish (which was more common until 1912 and remained in vernacular use, especially proverbs and slang). In that sense, his and Steiner's stories have much in common. Like all Jewish communities around the world, they were able to speak the native tongue of their country of residence, as well as other languages, including the localized Jewish dialect, which in Cohen's case was Ladino and in Steiner's case was Yiddish. Cohen's letters exhibit that linguistic variety often. Most letters were written in French but quite often, and especially during the war years, when there was a suspicion that an unfriendly person would read the letter, Ladino was used both as a more familiar form of communication and to hide sensitive information.

But unlike Steiner, that crucial and lifesaving second move is missing from the story of Leon Cohen and his family. How shall I begin the tale, the tale of the memory I did not have and yet possessed me?

The very first document in the Cohen Collection, the earliest testimony I have in front of me, is a note addressed to Leon Cohen on June 4th 1914, when he was only thirteen years old, from the *Profit Sportif Club*, acknowledging in Solitreo that he had been accepted into the club. The letter is signed off with a *Shalom* greeting and wishes young Leon success in his endeavour. Other items from that period that Leon had kept all those years and carried with him from Salonica to Paris are two receipts that Leon's father, Shabtai, received from the *Sportif Club* in Salonica, where he enrolled his son in two consecutive years.

Jumping ahead to 1923. Only three letters testify to what went on in Leon Cohen's life in 1923. All three describe an episode in his life that took place towards the end of the year. The letters concern his employment situation, a very important issue in those years in Europe that was still reeling from the devastation of the World War I that eventually led to the severe economic crisis of the late 1920s.

The first letter to start this narrative is dated November 14th 1923. He was twenty-two years old, still living in Salonica but had already been working since 1919 (when he was eighteen years old) for a commercial firm run by Richard Salem and Daniel Amar in Marseille, France.

Dear Leon,

I have just received a telegram from Mr Amar informing me that due to personal reasons, you will not be able to arrive in Marseille, as planned.

I have asked Mr. Amar to ask you to find a substitute for you, in case your arrival is further delayed. I truly hope your decision is only temporary. I would be very happy for you to arrive in

Marseille but of course I am unable to influence the personal circumstances that force you to stay in Salonica.

Still, and in the meanwhile, my very dear Leon, I understand that you will continue to work for Mr Pepo as our representative and during that time will oversee his book-keeping and his routine correspondence with the offices in Marseille. For performing these tasks, you will be awarded 1,500 francs each month. As I am aware that you have no other income. I have requested Mr Pepo to share with you a percentage of each deal you manage to bring to fruition.

If your decision to remain in Salonica is indeed final, please always feel free to consult with me if you decide to change employment.

Looking forward to hearing from you,
David Amar

Leon did not take long in responding. On November 30th, he wrote back. The fact that he kept a carbon copy, something he rarely did, shows the significance of the letter. The collection contains a few of Leon's letters, when he had chosen to make carbon copies. They are still a minority among the letters he received that he kept. Almost always the carbon copies are of letters regarding work. It is a common practice that mainly attests to Leon being an orderly and responsible professional. The letters he kept copies of were usually those that signified a turn of events or contained information he needed as a proof for later events. The string of the carbon copies, often printed on thinner paper, forms a special narrative in the collection. They alone represent Leon's genuine voice. As much as I wish he had kept copies of his more personal correspondence, this is the nearest we can get to know of his thoughts.

Dear Mr. Richard,

I have received and read your letter from the 22nd.

I cannot understand why you insist that I continue to work for Mr Pepo. I made it clear to Mr Amar that I have no such desire after I close your office here. Surely you can appreciate why I want to be independent. I have given this much thought and my decision is final. I have already informed you of my choice but agreed to stay with Pepo for a short time in order to bring to order the accounts with Marseille. I have set up a separate accounting system including all the transactions dealing with flour. Most of that work

*is already done, and once completed will be easily managed by
out-sourcing.*

*Quite a few very good firms have offered to employ me here.
I would not want to miss such an opportunity. I also have some
brokers who wish to work with me and of course there is always
the option of working free-lance. You know that I have to generate
a lot of income. That is why it is absolutely vital that I will stop
my contact with Pepo very soon. I can stay with him until the
end of December. That will give me enough time to tie up all
the necessary loose ends with Marseille and perhaps even find a
substitute. I will of course remain available to you to finish off all
matters relating to 1923.*

*I look forward to hearing from you as soon as possible. The delay
is making me ill.*

P.S.

*Please do not doubt the sincerity of my intentions. I am sure you
appreciate all the time and effort I have dedicated to your office
over the last three and a half years. I am sorry if that gave rise
to hopes that I will stay with you indefinitely. I must start on my
own path. I know that not working for you might be hard and I
will surely encounter hard times but I believe I will be successful
as I will as always work truthfully and honestly. Please do not put
any more pressure upon me to work for Mr Pepo and respect my
decision to go independent.*

Leon

A mere ten days later, on December 9th, Richard Salem replied.

Dear Leon,

*I was really surprised with the content of your letter. I hope it does
not really reflect your real feelings but is rather based on advice
that people gave you. I do not recognize the Leon I know in the
letter.*

*Of course, I cannot force you to work for Mr Pepo. I only
recommended that, having your best interests in my heart. I have
just written to him asking him to give you a raise in salary as well
as a percentage on deals completed. But still, if you think you can
get better terms elsewhere, or if you want to go free-lance, I will*

fully support you and not make it hard for you. I would not want you to hold anything against me in the future.

I offered you to come to Marseille with terms that, believe me, many young people would be thrilled to get. That was the spirit of my last telegram to Mr Amar. If you cannot come to Marseille due to familial circumstances, please do not hold that against me.

Having said all that, I would love to know what your plans are. If you want to get work through an agency, I can recommend some very good firms here that are still not represented in Salonica and suggest various strategies that might be beneficial. If I ever decide to settle in Salonica, which is certainly an option, you can rely on me that I will get you involved so that you benefit from it.

Finally, it is important for me that you know that I trust you wholeheartedly with our common interests in Salonica and any queries I might have. It is important that you remain open with me.

Looking forward to hearing from you.

P.S.

Without wanting to influence you in anyway, I still recommend that you do not leave Pepo's office before you have a solid alternative. Do not put yourself in the midst of something you may regret that concerns Pepo. I say this in total confidence and only for your own good. You know that I have no reason to favour Pepo's interests over yours.

Richard

What else took place in Salonica in 1923? What were the conditions that prompted young Leon to try and break away from what seemed like a good and steady position with his French patron?

There can be many answers to such a question. History can be told in many different fashions, often choosing one angle to emphasise a particular point of view. Is history really continuous as might seem from an external, seemingly objective point of view? Or is it episodic, showing only bit and pieces, leaving the gaps to be filled by our imagination and make-belief?

The year 1923, for instance, is the year Louis Armstrong (1901–1971) made his first recording with King Oliver's Creole Jazz Band in March, thus beginning a glamorous career that would only end nearly fifty years later in 1971. Marie Bonaparte, Freud's saviour in 1938, was yet to meet him. She was still in the midst of her search for love and sexual satisfaction. In her notebook of that time, optimistically entitled *The Happiness of Being Loved*, she wrote of her current love, the ailing but desperately in love Aristide Briand (1862–1932), who had been the French prime minster intermittently during those years.

She counted him as her seventh lover, who also gave her no reason to believe that she had been cured from her frigidity.

Spin the wheel again and you will see the marriage of Queen Elizabeth (1900–2002) to Prince Albert (1895–1952) (the future King George VI) in April of the same year. Nearly, a hundred years later, as I am writing this, her daughter, Queen Elizabeth II is still alive and well, having broken Queen Victoria's record of a living monarch. Nearer Salonica, on June 9th, a military coup in neighbouring Bulgaria ended Aleksandar Stamboliyski's (1879–1923) term as prime minister after four years. He was brutally tortured and murdered five days later by Macedonian terrorists. And all he did was try to suppress the nationalistic Macedonian movement but also stood against Mussolini's pressure to ally with Italy against the rising communist powers of Yugoslavia and Russia. In July, the Hollywood sign was inaugurated in California. Was there any awareness in either Bulgaria or California of the proximity of such disparate events? And for the duration of September, the Greek island of Corfu was occupied by Italian forces after the killing of an Italian officer. The occupation ended only as a result of the intervention of The League of Nations. In 1923, Lawrence Durrell, a writer without a home who was born in India to an Anglo-Indian family, was eleven years old. Next year, his father would send him to a boarding school in England in an attempt to make a proper British Gentleman out of him. Being sent away from his beloved Kim-world in India, would mark him for life, stamping upon his soul a secret and lasting sense of exile.

During the very same September, an earthquake in Japan killed an estimated 142,807 people; there was a military coup in Spain, the newspapers printers of New York went on strike and on the 29th, in Palestine, the British Mandate came into effect, officially creating the protectorate of Palestine as a homeland for the Jewish people under British administration.

A patent was filed in the USA for a television system by Vladimir K. Zworykin (1888–1982), who lived until 1982, long enough to see his vision become a universal reality, changing forever the entertainment habits of the whole population of the globe. Charlie Chaplin (1889–1977) made an untypical drama starring Edna Purviance, *A Woman from Paris*, W.B. Yeats (1865–1939) won the Nobel Prize for Literature after having previously been unsuccessfully nominated seven times.

And as the year draws to an end, on November 11th, Adolf Hitler (1889–1945) is arrested after leading the failed Beer Hall Putsch, only four days before hyperinflation in the Weimar Republic reaches its highest point.

And in Salonica? The scope of this book again only allows for a cursory review of the events that Salonica and its residents were subjected to during the first decades of the twentieth century. The economic and political situation has been unstable for decades. The bloody Balkan Wars of 1912–1913 have deprived the Ottoman Empire of many of its territories.[2] It had lost control of Salonica that was won by the Greek army, finally depriving both the Turks and the Bulgarians of their aspiration for the cosmopolitan city, a centre of trade and finance. It took quite a while for the Greek state to fully exercise its power in the city by its Hellenizing policies. The Muslim population of the city was deported, in exchange for the mass importation of Greeks from Asia Minor, by agreements capped by the Treaty of Lausanne. World War I and the Great Fire of 1917, which decimated the trade centre of the city, mainly Jewish, only increased the on-going crisis. In 1923, the Greek state tried to exclude Jews holding foreign passports from staying as part of the local Jewish community.[3] As in other cases of restrictions, local Jewish leaders were again successful in aborting such an initiative, which was part of an attempt to strengthen the independence of the Greek state.

For Leon Cohen, like many other young professional men, it was time for change and for independence. His older brother, Isaac, has left for France a few years ago, like many other men who were seeking their luck in the West. His father had died a few years ago. Along with his eldest brother, Henri, who was five years his senior, he had the responsibility of looking after his widowed mother and his younger brothers and two sisters, all yet unmarried and living at home. The young four ones were still teens. The youngest, Sam, merely twelve years old, had not yet had his Bar-Mitzva. So, any decision he was to take concerning his livelihood and place of residence affected not only him but also the rest of the family. As he wrote to Richard, he was under the obligation to generate income for his family.

As 1923 drew to a close, he was to remain in Salonica. But the seeds of the forthcoming move to France were sown and were even budding. I am left with a big gap – what were his thoughts? A young man of twenty-two years, what was he grappling with?

In the absence of his voice, I turn to the many doppelgänger voices I have gathered along my way, voices I had read, heard and imagined, voices that I will turn to on this postmemorial path as I try to make the ghost real.

Lawrence Durrell was twenty-three when he left his exile in England in 1935, his cultural homeland which he loathed, in search for his true voice. Durrell visited Paris during the time Cohen lived there. A possible meeting could have taken place.

Henry Miller (1891–1980), the American author, Durrell's mentor, was thirty-seven years old when he left his "air-conditioned nightmare" USA in search for his true voice in 1928. He will re-appear in my narrative in 1930. Suffice to say for now that the author of *The Tropic of Cancer*, which will scandalize Europe and North America in the late 1930s, lived in Paris during some of the time that Cohen did.

Both, like Leon Cohen, made Paris their first station on their journey that eventually brought them each to write literary masterpieces that had an impact upon many generations. Miller and Durrell were living in Paris during the very same years as Leon Cohen. Have they ever met? Did they cast their spell upon his soul as they have on mine?

Durrell, then. In *The Black Book*, published in 1938 after he had arrived in Paris to meet Miller, his mentor, he writes of his preparation for his journey that he is too preoccupied with the details but is certain to follow his own path, even though he feels mostly like a ghost. What matters is the journey.[4] Will he cross in that journey Leon Cohen's path, or is it all in my postmemorial imagination?

1924 – Planning the move to France

There are two 1924 documents in the collection. A whole year and only two pieces of papers to give evidence of the activities of Leon Cohen, his brothers, sisters and mother: 365 days with various comings and goings, meetings to keep, bills to pay, romances to maintain, promises to fulfil and dreams to frustrate.

The first is a letter from March from Richard Salem. Its content is surprising, considering what went on in the exchange of the previous year between the two when Leon indicated very firmly that he intended to cut loose from his business ties with Amar & Salem.

Dear Leon,

In your last letter, you asked me again whether I had any plans for you in Salonica and how I imagine your future.

You know that at the moment our firm has no interests in Salonica, not directly or indirectly, and that I am finally settled here in Marseille. Despite all my goodwill to help you, I cannot help you in Salonica. Nevertheless, and after much thought, and conversations with Mr. Amar, and in order to do you a favour that you would certainly appreciate, I decided to invite you to come to Marseille as my employee and pay you 800 francs a month. Apart from this salary, I will give you 4% of all the profits made in the office. You need to prepare yourself for the journey as soon as possible because we have other options and we want to complete our work team soon.

In order that there are no misunderstandings, I will raise the following points:

1   Your contract will be for two years.
2   You will carry travel expenses. I will however advance you the cost and it will be deducted from your future salary.

3   *You will have to provide yourself for all your living expenses in Marseille (food, lodging, etc.).*

If you agree to these terms, send me a telegram immediately with the word "agreement" and the date of arrival. You will also bring with you all the office documents that I left in Salonica, as well as the typewriter.

Best,
Richard

Trying to figure out what had taken place between November 1923 and March 1924 is like finding a missing piece of a puzzle that had been long lost. Leon's intention of becoming a free-lance accountant in Salonica seems to have been thwarted by the harsh economic reality of that time and he was forced to do what many of his generation did at the time – emigrate to a richer country where he hoped he could do better for himself.

The second of the two documents indicates that he had taken concrete steps towards re-establishing the trust that had existed between him and Amar & Salem. It is a notice of a contract signed between Richard-Daniel Salem and David-Solomon Amar on one side and Leon-Sabetay Cohen and Isaac Nadjari on the other side in the presence of the notary Louis Allegre.[5] The notice is published in the *Journal de Marseille, edition Judiciaire quotidienne (Daily Justice)*, published on an irregular basis between 1923 and 1955.

It is a legal contract that will be mentioned often in the coming years and gave quite a lot of concern to Leon. The contract states the founding of a subsidiary company under the auspices of the Salem & Amar firm, based in Marseille. Cohen and Nadjari are the directors of the company, which is given licence to trade food products for five years until 1931, in short – a grocery store. Amar & Salem are given powers of attorney to dissolve the new firm with ease while Cohen and Nadjari can only do so in case of death. It is a partnership of sorts, with Cohen contributing 5,000 francs, Nadjari contributing a shop he owns on 5 Cours Belsunce, Marseille and Amar & Salem, being the senior partners, bringing in the sum of 60,000 francs. That shop does not exist anymore, and its address points to a pedestrian area in the city, next to which a branch of *Société Marseillaise de Crédit* is situated today on 41 La Canebière. That address is today a tobacco shop. A quick walk westward, a mere six minutes away, will get you to Navette du Frioul where you can take a ferry to many destinations including the local international airport. Or, you could have received cargo shipped from across the Mediterranean. So, the Nadjari shop is no longer there, but one can easily appreciate its good location and proximity both to the commercial centre of the city and to easy access to cargos delivered by sea. So, a wise partnership? Was Leon Cohen *en route* to setting himself up in the company of successful tradesmen?

Emigration to post-World War I France was not uncommon. After the devastation it suffered and the reduction in the male workforce, France became the country with the highest rate of foreign population growth in the world in 1924.[6] France was becoming a nation of immigrants and by 1942, 11% of its population (more than five million people) were immigrants. And within that vast and diverse crowd, about 25,000 came from the Balkans, including Jews from Salonica. Despite growing anti-Semitism, and racism directed towards the Muslim immigrants from North Africa, they enjoyed relative security. France was being transformed by that immigration, enjoying unprecedented ethnic diversity as well as a sense of Mediterranean connectivity. The cities of Paris and Marseille developed into the focal points for the establishment of new shared commercial and sociocultural spaces. Though the dominant Jewish and Muslim immigrant communities found common ground thanks to their North African roots, Jews from the former Ottoman Empire territories, such as Greece, also formed closely knit familial, cultural and business connections. It is seemingly easier to trust someone from back home when one finds oneself in a new territory. As Leon Cohen had already good ties with Salem & Amar, it was only natural that it would be with them and other immigrant Salonica Jews that he had started his new life in France. That was true of Marseille where the majority of the Jewish community did not come from the Maghreb as in Paris, but from former Ottoman Empire countries. More than 60% of that community lived in the Port d'Aix neighbourhood where Leon bought the shop with Nadjari, just off La Canebière, Marseille's legendary central street, lined in the interwar years with numerous fashionable restaurants, hotels and cafés.

But, alluring as Marseille sounds with its cosmopolitan, buzzing cafés and restaurants, the promenade along the port, the fascinating multi-cultural encounters between Jews and Muslims, Leon was not destined to become part of that life. His journey took him elsewhere.

1925 – Turning a back on Marseille

How to summarize what during 1925 in Salonica and Paris without turning this study into an overwhelmingly detailed report? What stories are relevant in order for the memory to gain credibility and a sense of coherent narrative that would assist the reader in forming a subjective experience? Perhaps, the quest for a coherent narrative is a mistaken one; perhaps, the sense of randomness, so often present in human life, is more pertinent.[7]

Towards the beginning of November 1925, when he was nearly twenty-four years old, having left his mother's home in Salonica sometime during 1924 or early 1925, Leon wrote to his friend and business colleague Richard Salem in Marseille about his decision to finally stay in Paris. He had known Salem for several years as he was representing his firm in Salonica. The business co-operation consisted mainly of Cohen searching for retail business opportunities for Salem in Salonica and helping him with bureaucratic endeavours. Business was not good either in Marseille or in Salonica, and Salem was no longer able to provide enough work for Cohen in Salonica. He, therefore, urged him to come to Marseille where he would be able to employ him as an accountant on a more regular and secure basis. This was just based upon the business they had opened together in Marseille only a year earlier, on December 1924, consisting of a grocery shop owned by the firm Cohen had opened with Nadjari under the auspices of Salem.

He, therefore, must have been surprised to hear from Cohen in a letter from November 22nd sent from Paris that Cohen had no intention of returning to Marseille but planned to stay in Paris for the time being. Why did he change his mind and make a move that seemed to have more uncertainty than a promise? Was he such an adventurous character? Or did something happen after he travelled to Paris from Marseille that made it difficult to leave the glamourous city? Were family issues interfering with his business acumen?

Dear Richard,

As I am writing this letter to you, I am beginning to think of ways of recruiting staff for a new business enterprise. As I have already mentioned, my older brother Isaac has been in the advertisement business in Paris for some years now. Since the day he left Salonica his status was shaky. He had been waiting for an opportunity. Today, his business is thriving and we are in the process of starting several projects together. As you know, our family back in Salonica is not very happy. We are thinking of bringing all of them to Paris and mainly to find Rita a husband. Isaac has always wanted me to come and work with him but while I was still in Salonica I could not appreciate the scope of his business. Now that I am here, working alongside him and his wife, Martha, I can see the potential. It is a very unique enterprise here in Paris and it is something he made happen with his own hands. He has shown me how the business has developed over the last year. He needs me now more than ever since the intensive work has made him ill. He needs reliable and trustworthy partners. He has been paying some employees a lot of money since he could not take care of all aspects of his business due to his physical condition. He can no longer perform it all on his own. I really can't see how I can do anything else but stay by his side and help him the best I can.

You know I hold you in the highest esteem and you have always explained to me the importance of internship. I have worked for you for five years now and I have always done my best for you. But now I need to know that I can rely upon your support for what I am trying to achieve here in Paris. I hope and trust that you will understand me and be there for me.

Please consider all this carefully. I am awaiting your response with anticipation, Richard. I need your support.

Yours,
Leon

Leon's tone is that of a son to his father, asking for his approval as he sets out on an independent path that he worries will upset him. Five days later, on November 27th, Richard responded with mixed feeling. It is a warm letter but tinged with sadness and maybe even disappointment that again Leon turned down his genuine offers for help. Yet, he continues to hold a fatherly position, wishing Leon the best and continuing to offer him his support.

Dear Leon,

I must say that I was surprised by your strong desire to remain in Paris. There was no indication that you would do that when we last spoke, before you left. But as you know, I'm not indifferent to your circumstances. I place great value upon your future. So, even though your decision is inconvenient for me, I have no choice but to support your decision to stay in Paris, especially if you intend to bring your family over. I strongly recommend that you examine

*carefully this possibility, with all its implications, before you act
on it. So, I give you and your brother my blessing and hope that
your stay in Paris will not be indefinite.*

*I would appreciate it if you could come to Marseille next month.
We'll have time to discuss our business, and if your decision to
stay in Paris still holds, you will be free to go after you finish your
bookkeeping.*

Yours, Richard

Did Leon comply with Salem's request to arrive in Marseille by December
15th? It is impossible to tell from his letter of December 23rd.

Dear Richard,

*I have received your letter informing me that you have not yet
employed anyone and that you are thinking of calling me at the end
of the month in Marseille to arrange the accounts. I hope that since
you received my reply, you have been looking for an accountant
to do that work. I'm writing in the clearest possible way that I
will not be able to do the accounts for you this year. From what
I saw, even the balance of October is still unfinished. There is a
lot of work to be done, at least a month's work, and even though I
really want to help you, my schedule in Paris will not allow me to
be absent for so long. I will come to Marseille as soon as you hire
someone for your bookkeeping so that I can help and guide him for
a few days to do the work himself. Please understand.*

My best wishes to you and to Mr. David (Amar).

*Sincerely,
Leon*

Leon is quite clear about his intention not to travel to Marseille. Despite
their previous and present business connections and despite the warmth
that is still present in the tone of the letters, he is determined to follow up
his earlier resolve to break away from his connection with Richard Salem
and David Amar.

It is not an easy break, and it will take quite a while before all their mutual
interests are dissolved to their mutual satisfaction. The year 1925 is drawing
to a close, finding Leon in France as he had planned, but not in the warm
presence of his old business partners with whom he had been acquainted in
Salonica.

The address where Leon is residing at this time is 10 rue Richer, in the
Faubourg-Montmartre area, the fashionable Ninth arrondissement, only a

few blocks further along the road from the famous Folies-Bergères cabaret music hall, at 32 rue Richer. Still operational today as a tourist magnet, it was at its highest popularity during the very same years that Leon rented a small flat on that street. Was Leon a customer in that hall and the many entertainment businesses that filled that street? He was a single man, and judging from another string of letters he kept from that period, it is not hard to visualize him partaking in the celebrations.

To get an understanding as to why Leon found Paris alluring to the extent of turning down what seemed like a good offer from Marseille, I suggest turning to the American journalist Janet Flanner (1892–1978) who lived in Paris from 1925 until her retirement in 1975. In those fifty years, she wrote for *The New Yorker* magazine, reporting the various cultural happenings of the city. Those were exciting times. She wrote of the way each June the inexpensive Left Bank hotels began being booked up in advance for the whole summer by new Americans who would settle down for a couple of weeks there as if the quarter were a kind of summer resort and then pass on, full of memories and satisfactions. She describes Paris as a beautiful, alluring, satisfying city. It was a city of charm and enticement, to foreigners and even to the French themselves.[8]

Leon was not the only Greek Jew from Salonica who had found his way to the French capital in those years, hoping for a better future. The earliest indication of Greeks moving to France, mainly Paris and Marseille began with merchants in the second half of the nineteenth century. This commercial expansion was not solely limited to France but took place in all the major port cities of Europe, the Mediterranean and as far as Odessa, on the Black Sea. The Greek communities were successful in most cities they arrived at, even to the extent, in some historians' view, of re-kindling the *Great Idea* (*Megali Idea*), which, especially after the 1850s and 1860s and until 1922, inflamed a large part of the Greek diaspora; *The Great Idea*, mixing together memories of the Greek past from the classical, Hellenistic and Byzantine eras, aspired to the return of the young Greek kingdom to the geographical borders of the "Great Hellades" – the territories peopled by the Greeks, maintained under Ottoman domination as well as the lands where Greek civilization had exerted its influence in the past.[9]

Whether any of this was really a part of Leon's motivation and decision-making in regard to deciding where he was going to live is impossible to say. What is clear is that almost, if not all, of his correspondence in these years in France was with other Greek Jews from Salonica, like this letter from Nissim Mizrachi from Marseille, who wrote to him late in December. Nissim Mizrachi lived and worked in Marseille in Salem & Amar's firm. But he was not one of the managers of the firm and so his communication with Cohen was along different channels. He did not seem to be at all preoccupied with Cohen's decision to disengage from Salem & Amar and relates to Cohen in a very friendly manner, even providing him with information that might have helped Cohen to deal with the string of increasingly urgent telegrams that were beginning to arrive from Amar & Salem, requesting and then demanding his presence.

Dear Leon,

I'm sure you're really angry with me for leaving you so long without news. Trust me that I did everything in my power to find out information and share it with you, but nothing came up. I even went down to see Albert on Garibaldi Avenue (where Amar & Salem's offices were) and asked him to keep you updated. I hope he will. What is it that you are up to? Why are you staying in Paris? You know that Richard (Salem) is expecting you. He told me so many times. Has he written to you? If he hasn't, I think you need to take the initiative and write to him again. He is a good person but sometimes hard to understand.

Not much else is going on. I really miss your presence. The weather is really awful recently. Today is better. From what I heard, it is not so great in Paris either. Are you enjoying Paris? Getting to know it?

Waiting to hear from you.
Nissim Mizrachi

The family back home was just beginning to catch up with Leon's absence. A single postcard from Salonica that Leon kept stands alone as evidence. Eli, Leon's younger brother by five years, sent a postcard showing a photograph of young Solomon Matarasso.[10] The card is addressed to Leon, but the postal address given is Salem & Amar's office on 1 rue Venture, Marseille. On the back of the photo of Solomon, who looks caught off guard in the picture, Eli wrote:

I'm sending you a postcard of the cute Solomon. He seemed to be annoyed. I have received two letters from you, including the content in the envelopes (Money?). *I'll reply in more length tomorrow. We are very happy that you are progressing in your work and becoming more independent.*

At home everyone is fine. As in Marseille, the weather is very good and it hardly feels like winter. We received a postcard from Isaac and also wait still for a letter from him.

Yours,
Eli

Solomon, born in 1923, is two years old in the picture (see card on p. 24). He is Ines Cohen Matarasso's oldest child and the first grandchild in the family. This is Ines' first, but certainly not the last, appearance she makes in this tale. Her presence and importance will only increase with time and the developing familial events.

What had become of the Matarasso family? Solomon was twenty years old when the Greek police rounded up the Jews of Salonica on their way to their deaths in Auschwitz in 1943. Was his mother Ines with him? And his father Moise? And Moise's own Matarasso family, parents and siblings? His second daughter, Nelly, was seventeen at the time that the Nazi sent the Jews of Salonica to their death in 1943, and Rachelle was only four years old. None of them left any letters of their own. Their only memory is the very slim one captured by what Leon Cohen kept in the boxes (Figure 15).

In 1925, Solomon was still the only child of Ines and Moise Matarasso. Leon had only ever met him before his departure to France in 1925. He was informed of the new additions to the family by letters but was not able to

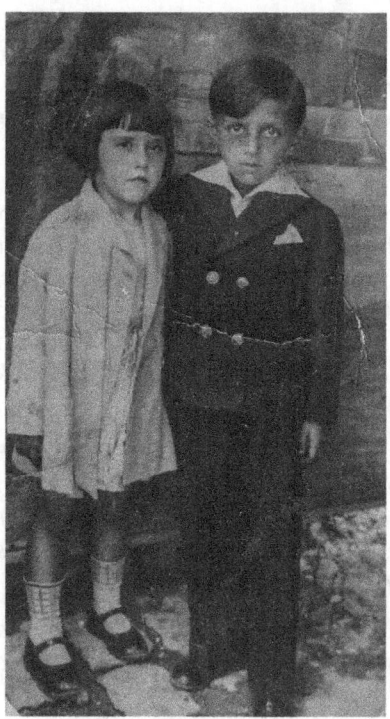

Figure 15 Solomon & Nelly Matarasso.

either see his nephews or enjoy their presence. These have become part of his terms of exile.

How to summarize what went on during 1925 in Salonica and Paris without turning this study into an overwhelmingly detailed report? What stories are relevant in order for the memory to gain credibility and a sense of coherent narrative that would assist the reader in forming a subjective experience? Perhaps, the quest for a coherent narrative is a mistaken one; perhaps, the sense of randomness, so often present in human life, is more pertinent.[11]

The year 1925, for instance, was the year that the building of the Monastirioton Synagogue, the official Salonica synagogue, was commenced. Finished two years later in 1927, it was the only synagogue the Nazis did not destroy, perhaps because it was used as a warehouse for the Red Cross during the occupation. Originally used as a religious centre for Jewish refugees arriving from the city of Monastiri, nowadays located in the Former Yugoslav Republic of Macedonia (FYROM, today North Macedonia) and named Bitola, a ghetto determined by Nazis forces in the densely populated Jewish Syggrou area before the eventual displacement of Jews in 1943. In later letters, we will see that it was indeed a place the Cohens visited.

The year 1925 was also the year that the initiative taken by the government of Alexandros Papanastasiou (1876–1936) bore fruit and the Aristotle University of Thessaloniki was founded, even though it took another year before it was actually opened. It was the same university that, after the destruction of the nearby Jewish Cemetery by the Nazis in 1942, expanded its grounds that were built over the desecrated burial area after the end of World War II. It took the Greek authorities until 2014 before a monument was erected on the grounds of the campus. Since then, that monument has continued to be a target for anti-Semitics attacks and has suffered great damage.

The third vertex in the Salonica-Paris-Tel-Aviv triangle, Tel-Aviv, is still dormant, as far as the Cohens are concerned. Having been occupied by the British and declared under mandatory rule in 1920, it was making its first step in the world as a new political entity. The Muslim population was still around 80% of the general population, which was reported to be around 700,000 people. The Jewish population was around 76,000, about 10% of the general population.

Though small, the Jewish community was busy, and in 1925, several significant events took place: February 6th saw the official opening of the *Technion, Israeli Institute of Technology*, which in a few decades would have as one of the students Shlomo Parenti, Rita Cohen's son. In the same year, another major academic institute opened, *The Hebrew University of Jerusalem*. The opening ceremony was attended by dignitaries such as Herbert Samuel (1870–1963), the first nominally practising Jew to serve as a Cabinet minister in Britain and to become the leader of a major British political party, who was appointed to be the High Commissioner of Mandate Palestine from 1920 to 1925. Sigmund Freud was asked to be the president of the University and turned it down, a job taken up by Haim Weizmann (1874–1952), who was one of the founders of the University. Freud was proud to be a Governor of the University, alongside Martin Buber (1878–1965) and Albert Einstein (1879–1955).

1926 – On brotherly love and young men in France

How did Leon make his way from Salonica to Marseille? 1,477 kilometres separate the two cities. Today, there are several possible routes: by plane, train, ferry or car. A direct flight would take about four hours. Though there was an airfield in the city built during World War I, it was only used for military purposes. There were no international flights from Salonica until 1938, so it was not by plane that he had left his birthplace. What route did he take? Where did he stop along the way? Whom did he meet? Questions, unanswerable questions.

The letters of 1926 indicate a very busy year. A very lively exchange of letters between Leon in Paris and friends in Salonica and Marseille as well as business interactions slowly forming and shaping Leon's future as an accountant. Leon seemed busy both maintaining and utilizing old contacts to make his way in his new home, as immigrants tend to do, as well as making new contacts that will help him to establish himself independently away from home. Throughout 1926, he seems to be both holding on to the hope of bringing the rest of his family from Salonica to the "New World" of France, and at other times considering going back home. His sense of being an exile is slowly taking shape.

The letters can be grouped thematically into those dealing with his business interactions with Salem & Amar in Marseille, letters aimed at developing new business contacts both in France and in Salonica and letters from his Salonica friends, some of whom live in Marseille, who keep him updated both about the happenings in Salonica as well as the prospects of staying in France. Thus, Leon's place of exile in France bears very strong connections to his home, acquiring more and more a sense of being both familiar and strange, *an unheimliche* kind of existence.

A flurry of telegrams sent from an increasingly perplexed Richard Salem from Marseille filled the first few months of 1926. Richard is still urging Cohen to come to Marseille in order to complete the accountancy for 1924 and to deal with the management of the shop that they bought together on 5 Cours Belsunce.

The fact that Leon kept those telegrams must mean that he took them seriously. But he did not seem to respond to them. Richard seems to be puzzled and upset by this. It is unlike Leon to treat his benefactor like that, who treated him as a friend and not only an employee and a business associate.

A letter from January 6th throws some light on the matter.

Dear Sirs,

I take the liberty to write to you on behalf of my brother Leon.

He had written to you after arriving in Paris about his plans and the projects he started with me. He also wrote that he would no longer be able to do your bookkeeping.

You have repeatedly asked him to come to Marseille, despite his clear statement that he will not be doing that. I think Leon did all that he was supposed to for you. Since my own interests are connected to his, I am really bothered that you expect him to be at your disposal. You will have to stop that. I suggest that you do all that is necessary to relieve him of any obligation he supposedly has towards you.

He also shared with me the situation he is in with you, regarding the grocery store. It is not without surprise that I have heard all this. I hope that you were planning to be fair with my brother, with whom I now share a company, regarding the profits that you expect from your venture. I would like to know about those profits as soon as possible. I think that if my brother is an employee of yours, you must give him higher profits than anyone else.

So, if you want to contact Leon, I expect you to do that on this account and let me know, as his partner and brother, the exact situation and what profits my brother is getting.

Please do not be alarmed by my letter. I have decided to write to you directly and not via my brother, only because I look after the future of our family.

> *Looking forward to your response.*
> *Isaac Cohen*

With this letter, Isaac, Leon's older brother, the one who had left their home in Salonica a few years before him, enters the stage and occupies his unique place. Isaac's character is prominent in the collection, mostly due to his reluctance to answer letters from his family, as will be revealed in years to come. This is the longest and most detailed letter from Isaac in the whole collection. Future communications are brief and mainly concerned with information about his whereabouts and requests, sometimes desperate, for financial aid.

The tone of the letter that Isaac allows himself to use deserves some consideration. Presuming he did not have prior contact with Salem, it can be read as quite an offensive letter. Taking into consideration that Salem was a father figure for Leon makes the offence even greater. It can perhaps be seen as an attack upon patriarchal authority, an attack Leon himself was loathed to make and thus split that part off, projected it onto Isaac, thus appointing him, consciously or not, to execute what he, Leon, could not bear to do.[12]

Isaac was three years older than Leon. He left Salonica before Leon, but there is no record as to when exactly and in what circumstances. What was the relationship between the brothers in Salonica before Isaac left?

The letter Isaac wrote to Salem & Amar in Marseille shows how deeply he has become involved in Leon's affairs at that early period of Leon's stay in France. It is a letter written in patronizing terms, assuming that Leon had to be protected and guided as if he were a helpless child. Seeing Leon's grimacing face in the family photograph, it is possible to speculate that perhaps that was Isaac's impression of his younger brother.

The letter Leon himself wrote to Salem & Amar a few days later, on January 18th, which must have been written before he had seen the letter they had written in response to Isaac's letter, though far gentler and more conciliatory, justifies such a view of the brothers' current relationship. By that time, Leon was already using a letterhead carrying the name of the new firm he had established with his brother Isaac – *Comptoir Industriel des Manufactures & Usines Réunies*, located at Leon's home address at 10–12 rue Richer.

Dear Mr. Richard

I haven't had any news from you. My brother told me he wrote you a letter and told me that he was surprised to not receive any answer from you. He thought that the change in our business relationship should be documented. Since you and I have no more common business, it's clear that the business on Garibaldi Avenue (the grocery shop, R.A.) should be finished with. Please do whatever necessary to make it so.

As I have tried several times to respond to your requests to set a date for my visit to Marseille to settle our business and you have not responded, I believe that I have fulfilled my duties towards you. Nevertheless, because of my personal relationship with you over the last six years I have worked with you, and because of the respect I have for you, I can still come to Marseille for twenty days and maybe even a month if you feel you need my help. We could at the same time settle all questions regarding the shop on Garibaldi Avenue.

Yours Sincerely,
Leon

The surprised, perhaps resentful but still civil and business-like Salem did not take long to respond to Isaac's letter. Addressing the letter to Leon at 10 rue Richer, he wrote a response signed both by him and his partner David Amar.

Dear Sir,

We have received the letter from your brother and we are surprised by the questions he is asking about the grocery shop. Please convey to him yourself all the necessary information, as we do not really understand why he asks us these questions.

We thought that you had postponed your arrival in Marseille because your brother is ill so you could have only come here "for a few days to give your replacement the necessary information". Well, we don't need that anymore because we've already organized the bookkeeping.

Now we ask that you return to us the key to your safe. Please tell us how much was in the safe on your departure day. According to the bookkeeping, the amount was 549 francs (about 300$ in today's currency). *The expenses recorded under the small fund are 177 francs. That means the amount of the remaining amount is 372 francs.*

We wish you all the best of luck again with your business.

Regards,
Amar & Salem

Salem & Amar wrote the second letter of response on February 27th, this time a direct response to Leon's own letter from January.

Dear Sir,

We have received your letter and we are surprised at your intense desire to get rid of your business on 60 Boulevard Garibaldi. We do not understand the reasons why you are doing so. You know the kind of work we do is completely risk-free. If it is the fiscal matter that is bothering you, please recall that our accounts show a profit of around 10,000 francs, so that your profit stands at 5% which is 560 francs. We pay all taxes.

We hope we will not be forced by your decision to change the ownership of the shop and sell your part in it, as this will incur very high costs for us. In addition, if you really insist that we transfer the business to someone else, we will in turn have to ask you to give us back the money you owe us right away as well as the amount left at the safe on the day you left Marseille. We don't believe you want to do all that.

We very much regret the attitude and tone you have adopted since leaving the office, and we do not think there is any justification for that because we have always been exemplary with you.

Regards,
Amar & Salem

Richard was not the only business contact Leon was jeopardizing on account of his ill-fated partnership with Isaac. In a letter dated February 27th, he turned down an offer from an old Salonica acquaintance, Haim, from whom he received an invitation to become the representative of a firm named M. Sasson & Gie, rue Vasilleos Heraclios in Salonica. The offer contained a request to receive Leon's conditions as well as his areas of expertise. It promised that if all went well, Leon would be entrusted with dealing with large-scale orders. Initially, Leon turned down the offer on the grounds that he had just entered the advertisement business with his brother. He did, however, keep the door open for the future in case he found the advertisement business not to his liking, as indeed happened quite soon. He made sure to write the letter in a very warm style, not neglecting to pass on his best regards to Mr. Solomon Hasson, the go-between, and his parents from Salonica. It was indeed a wise move as will soon become apparent.

It did not take Leon long to realize that turning down the offers from Salonica and Marseille was a mistake, as is shown by his response to Salem & Amar when he replied on March 19th.

Dear Sirs,

I received your February 27 letter and I am very saddened by your impression of my intentions. Still, if you think the tone of my letters has offended you in some way, I hope you believe it was not my intention. I am very sorry and deeply apologize.

I have no intention of being disrespectful to you, I will always be grateful for all that you have done for me. I will never forget that you have always been excellent employers.

As for the Garibaldi business, I certainly do not want to create unnecessary expenses by transferring the ownership but instead will wait until the shop is closed. Please do not regard this as distrust on my part. And if you want to keep the shop going, I will take care of it very seriously and I am sure I will achieve very good results. I ask that you consider my offer so that you will see it as a sign that I am coming towards you.

I cannot go into further details in this letter but I can only say that I will neither stay in Paris nor work with my brother. Before I make my final decision and maybe go back to Salonica, I will definitely share my thoughts and consult with you.

Back to our common interest, I think we can work together unless you no longer trust me, which I hope isn't the case. I am sure it is wiser at this stage to continue our joint business, even if only for a limited time, and then sell it when the time is right to maximize our profit.

I have realized that the advertising business doesn't suit me and I feel better with the kind of transaction we deal with, selling coffee etc. However, I do not regret the three months that I have spent in Paris, which I found very interesting, in every way. I truly hope I have not jeopardized your confidence.

Looking forward to hearing from you soon.

Leon

P.S.

If you think a phone call is needed, please let me know and I will do that.

A serious breach of trust between Leon and Isaac brought Leon back to his senses and prompted him to amend his connection with Salem. What was it with which Isaac tempted Leon by setting up their advertising firm, a firm that has left no trace whatsoever in the *Bottin*[13] professional register in Paris at that time? Leon has obviously realised within a very short period of time, between January and March, that he had better stick with the known and familiar rather than go into one of Isaac's ventures. Only time will tell just how right he was.

Salem & Amar responded in a letter from March 29th, addressed to Leon's new address on 96 Rue Doudeauville in the 18th Arrondissement, where he seems to be lodging with a Mme Henc. The flat is a mere eight minutes' walk from Basilique du Sacré-Cœur. So, Leon not only ended his short-lived business association with his brother but also moved, two kilometres away from his first Parisian lodging. The 18th Arrondissement, also known as Butte-Montmartre, is located on the right bank of the River Seine made famous for its artistic nature due to some well-known residents. For instance, Pablo Picasso (1881–1973) lived a few hundred meters away from Leon's flat until 1918. Was Leon aware of that? Did it have any bearings upon his life? I can imagine him walking in the evening the steep streets of Montmartre, watching the people mill about. Were his thoughts concerned with art, or was he too preoccupied with the daily and mundane hardships of a young Greek immigrant in a city that was perhaps exciting for him but was also opaque? Knowing the language was certainly an advantage. The very few photos he had taken of himself in those years showed that he had a suit. He also had a business card printed for him. What were his thoughts? How angry was he with Isaac for letting him on a wild goose chase that had cost him his job and almost his friendship with his benefactor Salem? Did he write back home to Salonica about all that, or was he sparing them the knowledge that Isaac was off track again?

In April, Richard Salem wrote back, a kind of a wake-up call to Leon.

Dear Sir,

I am sorry we could not respond to your letter sooner as we have been very busy. We were glad to see that you still want to keep your interest in our firm.

We are fully aware that at the beginning of your stay in Paris, you had your moments of doubt. It was clear from your writing and the general nervous atmosphere you generated. We fully understood that it was about personal issues and the people who influenced you back then. We will not let all that adversely affect our opinion of you, especially now that we see that your commitment to us has not changed at all.

You write that you are ready to return to Marseille to work for us in order to follow a business plan to develop the Garibaldi store with some new initiatives so that the profits of this business are increased. We believe you are sincere in your intentions, but we are sorry to say that we have other plans for the store. As you know, our plan was to close the store eventually, which we have been trying but still to no avail. We are now stuck with old stock which we don't believe we can sell. On top of that we have high overheads and almost zero profits.

Regarding our Rue Venture office. After you left, we've been helped by Albert to work for us, and at his family's request, we raised his salary and made him our accountant. So despite all our good will towards you, we are really sorry to have to turn down your offer to return to Marseille and work with us.

We did have an idea that we might introduce you to our associates at Mizrachi company to help them with their coffee trade as a broker, but after further consideration realizsed that because of the recent big crisis in the markets, brokers are not earning enough so you will be really hard pushed to make ends meet. You see, we look after you.

However, and since we really care for you, we offer the following: At Franses Fils, 15 Rue d'Hauteville, in Paris, they are looking for a good accountant and they have even written to us to know if you are available. You may approach Sam Franses and offer them your services.

Besides, there's also the Aelion & Ezratty business which just started on Rue du Faubourg-Poissonnière, by the Bergère telephone company. You can contact Isaac and Sam Aelion from Salonica who are the owners in partnership with J. Ezratty, Hasday Ezratty's brother. We think this business also needs an accountant, so maybe you can work for both companies to make a profit.

In any case, let us know what you do and what your plans are, we would love to know if any of this is successful.

We are waiting to hear from you,

Regards,
Amar and Salem

Amar & Salem's concern for young Leon is moving. Being businessmen, they did move on and managed without him, but also would not abandon a native Salonican and offer him real advice and direction for him to pursue. They are very sensitive and gentle regarding Leon's relationship with Isaac, which clearly had cost him his position with them. They bear no grudges, perhaps because of old ties back home and perhaps because they themselves were familiar with Isaac and his antics and therefore did not blame Leon for the temporary lack of judgment regarding his decision to break up with them.

Leon must have followed their advice and approached Sam Franses, who in April made inquiries with Salem about the salary that was expected of him to pay Leon. Richard wrote to Leon informing him that he had told Sam that his monthly salary was 1,400–1,500 francs (about $1,000 in current value), which was then just around the average wage for a professional. A loaf of bread cost about half a franc in those days, a pound of meat cost about 3 francs, an average rent would be around 300 francs a month, so Leon's wage was probably enough to live on, perhaps even allowing him to put some aside for saving or to send back to his family in Salonica without difficulties. Leon was, of course, grateful for the information and informed them he had indeed contacted both firms, as suggested.

Once an understanding was agreed upon between Leon and his former employers in Marseille, the selling of the shop could go forward. It still took several months and quite a few telegrams until the correct Power of Attorney was sent and the shop was closed. Leon did not hide his relief in a late May letter, which he addresses to Richard Salem at his 105 Avenue du Prado address.

Dear Sirs,

... I am very pleased to know that you have finally sold the business on Garibaldi Boulevard. I have to admit I'm glad the business is no longer in my name. Even though I trust you completely, I am glad I will not have to think about it anymore, as I'm busy all day in my new job. Please send me all the necessary paperwork so I can add my signature where it is required. And then please pass me a copy of the papers showing the liquidation of the business.

Yours,
Leon Cohen

Around the same time, a new connection with Salonica was made, which perhaps helped Leon in his decision to end his venture with Isaac. On March 13th, Benico Segura, an old friend, writes to Leon, still at a time when Leon was considering returning to Salonica, as shown in his correspondence with Nissim and other Salonica friends who have themselves migrated to France during the year. Benico's letter shows in its intimacy, the close relation he had with Leon.

Very dear friend,

I have received the letter sent from Paris, or more precisely the one that you wrote in Paris on February 25, and it arrived only on March 12. Which means that after you wrote your letter, you either wanted it to experience the soft fabric of your vest or that Paris-Salonica communications are not very good. All this to tell you that your letter arrived very late.

Well, let me get to the point. I saw your mother this morning. I thought she was pretty sad, missing her dear Leon, whom she really wanted by her side.

As you know, we are in the middle of an economic crisis. I cannot deny that our even our own business is currently undergoing a major crisis and the lack of activity of the business sector is quite critical. But your mother, who is thinking of her love for you before all, is sure that with your kindness, together with your nature, active, smart and strong capabilities, you will find work very easily here. I also think like her. So, because I am well acquainted with the opportunities of the Salonica scene, I do not think that for a moment you will have any trouble finding a good job. The crisis does not concern the best of us.

*I understand you're working with... (*unclear...*). So I wonder why you need to extend your stay in Paris. You lack money, you are busy with a business that does not really interest you, and even if you succeed one day, you have to say goodbye to your brother (that is the spirit of your letter). I do not understand why you are staying in Paris. Instead of wasting your time in a business that seems to me that it won't work out anytime soon, instead of putting yourself in the Paris office, isn't it better for you to come back? The crisis, yes. But I repeat, it will never be bad enough to leave you without work. Even taking into account that you will earn little here, your needs will be met, and most importantly, you will help your mother who cannot live in such an uncertainty for much longer. She is caught in between longing for you and on the other hand waiting for your help from Paris. Such help will probably take many years before it takes any real shape.*

I think I explained myself very well and I am sorry for getting too involved but you did invite me to do so in your last letter. That's why I am writing as if you are my brother, heart to heart.

As for the political situation, it is clear and transparent to you. Attached you will find information on the subject that should ease your mind if you wish to return.

I must point out that all I am saying is not because of what your mother feels. My argument for your return is based upon careful calculations which I have also double checked with Nissim Mizrachi and Isaac who are currently in the office with me, as I type these lines, and agree with me completely.

Let me know what you decide to do. Be open and share all your thoughts with me, even the most intimate ones and we will both try to find a solution to the problem together.

You can count on my absolute discretion,

Benico

As is already known, Leon decided to stay in Paris. His hesitation was most likely due to the complexity raised by the attempted, and failed, joint business venture with his brother Isaac. Once he got over that, he showed that he indeed possessed the firm character that his friends believed he had and put his mind to strengthening his position in France. No doubt, he still had in mind the interests of his family and sensed that in France, he would be in a better position to support them through the hardship they were going through in Salonica. Having apparently turned down Benico's offer, he wasted no time and took on new business opportunities, as is evident from a letter he received from Benico's brother, Leon Segura. Writing from his Salonica office which deals in Affaires Théâtrales, presumably an agent for projectors and similar equipment, Leon Segura writes on April 11th.

Dear Mr. Cohen,

With the recommendation of my brother Benico Segura, I request that you make contact with the Pathé Consortium Cinema, 67 Rue du Faubourg Saint-Martin, and order for me the spare parts of the Pathé projector, with the specifications which you will find included in the order.

I have deposited the necessary funds, 250 francs, in account no. 253019/151947 at Westminster Foreign Bank in Paris. Please send us the goods as soon as possible in two or three shipments. There is no need to tell Pathé that this order is for Greece.

Thanks in advance,
L. Segura

Leon's decision to remain in Paris is welcomed in Benico's next letter from Salonica on April 30th.

Dear Leon,

I received your 10th letter, which I awaited impatiently.

I was glad to read that you found a job that allows you to earn well, even more glad to hear that you want to move your relatives to France. Most important is that your dear mother will not have to live alone. That you will be together, in Salonica or France. For her it will always be great happiness. Naturally, your project to move your family to France has many benefits. First of all, you already have a good job, as you say. In addition, it would be good for your dear ones to be able to leave the unstable atmosphere of Salonica.

Since I am very busy, I did not have a minute to visit your dear mother. But I am sure she is very happy about the development and her upcoming move to Paris, near her dear Leon. It was your brother Benjamin, whom I met a few days ago and with whom I exchanged a few words about you, who told me with much enthusiasm that you seriously think to move everyone to France.

It is clear that your project cannot happen overnight. So I ask that you keep me informed of all your intentions.

I am glad that you have been contacted by my brother Leon and I hope that your transactions with him will be beneficial.

Isaac and Nissim send their regards. I'd rather send you a kiss and wait for the news from you.

P.S.

Sorry I typed this letter with a machine. My fingers are no longer used to writing with a pen and ink. You will only need to see the 6 letters of my name in my handwriting.

My brother Leon, who received your letter from the 20th, asked me to pass you some additional instructions concerning his order.

He said that you don't have to go yourself to get the items he asked for. You can instead send a letter to Pathé, 67 Rue du Faubourg Saint-Martin and ask for the prices of those items, and then send them the amount so that they can be sent to you by mail. The reason why my brother didn't place the order directly with Pathé in Greece is because they have a representative that my brother doesn't want to deal with.

With thanks and apologies.

Regards,
Benico

A letter from Leon Segura on June 6th confirms that the new contact Leon made in Salonica is proving successful and despite various delays in delivery due to the Greek postal service, business is going well. Leon has found a client in Salonica that he can work for. Now that his partnership with Salem & Amar is liquidated, he is free to turn to new horizons.

It seems that Leon's quick recovery of his senses served him well in other old contacts he had with Salonica. Though the opportunity with the Sassons did not materialize, it was not entirely lost. Haim made another attempt, this time asking him for help as he himself was on the verge of moving from Salonica to France. Realizing Leon was no longer in Marseille and presumably interpreting that as progress, he wrote on February 21st, showing both a potential for business as well an intimacy with Leon well beyond business.

Dear Leon,

Perhaps the last letter I sent you to Marseille didn't reach you. I now realise you are no longer there!

Here we are going through very difficult economic times. All businesses are stuck and no one can tell when and how we can emerge from this crisis that feels as if it has been going on for several centuries.

I know that in France the situation is not good either, but certainly not worse than here. The difference being that the French currency is stronger since there is more import.

I asked you in my last letter to help me as much as you can with connections with France. Among other things, we are interested in the import of black, white or red wool. We are also interested in other products but at the moment we want to concentrate on wool which is always in good demand.

With each offer sent to us, a sample is needed and the price should be listed for each net pound. Our commission is 3%. The shipping cost should be included. We will pay 50% in advance and the rest once the cargo arrives.

I hope, dear Leon, that you can make this happen and I assure you that you can also get something from this.

I understand that you did not find Marseille chic enough so you are now among the Parisians. But you need to get rid of that chilly Salonica attitude if you want to get anywhere. I know that making small talk is hard for you but you will have to learn to do it.

A big hug from me,
Haim

The next letter from Haim, on March 22nd, arrived in Leon's hands soon after the crisis involving Isaac and Amar & Salem was over. Leon presumably wrote back to Haim, telling him that his partnership with Isaac was over. He must have been in a very low place after the break-up, having lost both his job in Marseille and the prospects of the joint venture with Isaac. From Haim's letter, it is clear that in March 1926, Leon was contemplating admitting that being in France was not working out as expected and he was planning to return to Salonica.

Dear Leon,

Your letter from the 16th is in my hand, and I am very sorry to hear about the set-back in your plans. I would of course love to see you again in Salonica, so I will try and answer all your questions:

1   *Military service. There is no tax (bedel-i eskeri) to pay. I am not sure whether they will want to conscript you. The situation is unstable.*
2   *The financial situation is very bad.*
3   *The political situation from a Jewish point of view: In my opinion, it is usual, as of now.*
4   *Business situation is not brilliant. Don't be over-optimistic. It is not just a matter of hard work. A lot of luck is involved.*

So, I hope this gives you a clear and accurate picture of the state of affairs here, as you asked me to. If you do decide to come back, you will need to follow closely on all developments.

Before you come back and if you are able to do so, you need to personally reach out to important exporters and importers of any kind so that you can attain representative status with them. Don't turn down any offer and seize whatever business is offered. We will be able to use the connections you will make to both our benefits. You can always rely on me.

I don't want to write jokes to you because I'm guessing your appetite for humour is limited.

So, I am now anxious to hear from you.

Yours,
Haim

Haim's news bulletin is very illuminating. Did it provide Leon with the necessary information to help him consider his options and not just rush to return to Salonica on the rebound of the failed venture with Isaac?

Military conscription for Jews in Greece was an important issue. Serving in the army, as Jews did during World War I, was an important part of the Jewish community's effort to show involvement and loyalty to the Greek state, which became the new sovereign of the city in 1912. But it was not an uncommon practice for some Jews to try and avoid the service on religious or other grounds. In 1926, the Jews were neither expected to serve nor pay the tax, *bedel-i askeri*, that had allowed them to be exempted collectively from military service in the past.[14]

The collection holds two photographs of Leon's father, Shabtai, in military uniforms. So, the Cohens did have a tradition of serving in the army, a tradition kept years later by Leon's younger brothers Sam and Dino, who may well have joined the Jewish resistance movement during World War II.[15] Haim mentions two people in relation to military service. The first, Benico Segura, Leon's friend and someone who helped him make business connections in Salonica. The second reference is to Isaac. Did Haim tell Leon to discuss the issue of military service with Isaac since that was the reason Isaac left Salonica, to avoid conscription? And was that part of the reason Leon himself left? And if so, was that something that was not to be mentioned in letters?

Haim's description of the political and economic situation in Salonica tallies with other reports. Not only was Salonica still recovering from the devastating damage the big fire of 1917 caused but also dealing with a second blow. In 1922, as part of the peace negotiations held at Lausanne, the Greeks and Turks agreed to exchange populations. More than a million refugees were directed to Macedonia and Salonica, putting an unbearable pressure on the city's already shaken infrastructure. As most of them were Orthodox Christians and to allow them to better their economic position, market day was changed from Sunday to Saturday, causing a nearly lethal blow to the Jewish commercial community, which until then dominated the city's economy. It was considered an official anti-Semitic measure. The Jewish community had to adapt quickly in order to survive by observing the Sabbath only in part and sacrificing some of it to maintaining a business in the markets. As would transpire in later years, the Cohen family itself kept struggling. In 1926, four of the Cohen children were still living at home: Rita, twenty-four years old, was working as a teacher at *Alliance Israélite Universelle*, as was Benjamin, aged twenty-one, and Eli, aged twenty. Dino, aged seventeen, and Sam, aged fifteen, were still at school, which was increasingly costly. Sustaining the family could not have been an easy task for widow Rachelle.

Henri, the eldest brother, thirty-two years old, married and soon to father his firstborn, Shabtai (b. 1927), and Ines, married and a mother of Solomon, three years old, were living independently, but as the letters show, were quite often without enough means. Therefore, Leon's thoughts about returning to Salonica without having made a fortune were met with hesitation on Haim's side. He gave Leon sound advice that if he did decide to return, he must capitalize on the contacts he was able to secure while still in France.

The allure of Paris for young Salonican men as a place where one can escape one's problems is also evident in another letter from Haim, who was still in Salonica. Leaving one's motherland at a time of crisis is an option taken by many who could. Haim seems to be in such a position as he writes on April 20th, a very warm letter, which shows the level of intimacy he shared with Leon.

Dear Leon,

I was glad to read in your letter from the 10th that you would soon have a new job with such a salary that would allow you bring your dear family to Paris.

It's been a while since I opened my heart to you. You know me well and how important it is for me to share the good and bad moments of my life.

I am at a low ebb right now. Ever since I lost my mother six months ago, I have been very sad. I hope you won't be angry with me for hiding it from you until now. I did try to hide this weakness and it took a little courage to write this.

In this difficult moment of my life, I learned many things. These experiences only reinforced my nihilistic nature. You can't imagine how unbearable life has become. The atmosphere here is really making me sick. I would give a few years of my life to get out of Salonica, to make a change in me, even if very minimal.

Last time we wrote to one another about your possible return here. I told you about the economic crisis we are going through here, even worse than in France.

Will you think I'm crazy if I talk to you again about wanting to come to Paris? It is my strongest wish and getting stronger even if I will have to pay a heavy price. And that's why, dear Leon, when you write to Benico "I hope someday you will all join me here, because I know how Benico and Henri will be happy in France," you're just reinforcing this fire that is slowly destroying me, rather than calming it down. I think if I make a move, they will join me.

You write to us that you want to bring your dear family over. If that happens, my problem will be already partially solved. I won't have to look after them anymore. That is, if you all agree that I will be part of the family and help me with my daily needs. Please put some thought into it.

That's all I have to write to you. Please do everything you can to help me. I have no family obligations here so I can act independently. I hope to hear from you soon. Benico send his love.

Haim

Who was Haim, apart from being Leon's friend? From another letter written soon after the last one, he urges Leon to complete the selling of the shop on Garibaldi Boulevard as soon as possible. He must have been, then, involved in some way with Amar & Salem but wrote to Leon as a friend, seeking to look after his best interests. As proof of that, he sent Leon a list of firms in Paris he believed could provide him with just the networking needed to establish himself as a representative, regardless of whether he stayed in Paris or returned to Salonica. He always signed his letters with his first name only, so it will remain another mystery, another lost ghost.

The next letters from Haim indicate that he has moved from Salonica to France, as it was sent from his new address, 95 Boulevard National, Marseille, on July 20th, conveying his worries. Haim is a dedicated letter writer, sharing thoughts and feelings. His letter is a window into the mind of a young man in the 1920s. Interestingly, many of his preoccupations and observations seem relevant in 2020, a century later...

My dear Leon

... I have to apologize for my prolonged silence.

... business is not so hot. It's been a hard year in industry. Reduced orders, customers not paying on time. Add to that the difficulty in getting credit and there you have the whole messy picture...

... I see Nissim often and he also complains about the crisis. Sadly, this is the situation of our times. Everybody is just looking out for themselves, without thinking too much about their neighbour. That's the hardest thing, because with a little collaboration, a lot could have worked out better. But we will not be able to change the century's mentality, which is based on money and selfishness. We are among the happy ones because we still have honest friends. Everything else is emptiness.

But let's leave philosophy aside. I want to tell you that I have found love in Grasse. Another two in Marseille and one in Morocco... Having said that, I can imagine what you think of me and if you write to me every now and then, I am the happiest man.

I kiss you,
Haim

Capturing the spirit of the times, Haim delivers a message of existential despair fashionably mitigated with a turn towards physical love and lust, reminiscent of the writing of several authors who lived in Paris. For instance, the times were experienced as tough indeed, as is apparent from another

July letter written by someone from a different circle altogether, James Joyce (1882–1941).

It is far too hot and the franc having fallen to 150 has jumped back to 192 in four days… I certainly have a capacity for work but I wish I had more agility and imagination… I have been for years staring at an old print of the sacrifice of Cain and Abel and it is only a week ago that it struck me how tactful it was of Abel to slit the throats of the firstlings without any divine injunction as yet to kill the Cains of the flock.[16]

Would Leon have answered in a similar vein? Were those the issues that were preoccupying him? Joyce and his family lived at nineteen different addresses during the decades he stayed in Paris. When writing that letter, he was recovering from one of his many eye operations and was wearing the famous eye patch, captured in the photograph taken that year by Berenice Abbott (1898–1991), the American photographer who was also living in Paris during those years and who took an active part in the Parisian avant-garde photography scene of those times that included Man Ray (1890–1976), André Kertész (1894–1985) and Eugène Atget (1875–1927). Joyce himself was living at 2 Square Robiac, on the other side of the Seine from Leon at 96 Rue Doudeauville. Was Leon aware of the existence of the author of *Ulysses*, only a few kilometres away? Could they have come across one another in one of Joyce's regular haunts such as Shakespeare & Co. bookstore at 12 Rue de l'Odeon where the owner Sylvia Beach (1887–1962), Joyce's benefactor reigned? Or perhaps he could have run into him at Les Trianons restaurant on the Boulevard Montparnasse, a place Joyce frequented, seeking to avoid the popular places where the chic artists roamed, which was only a few hundred metres from Leon's flat. Both were equally without means in those years.

Once in Marseille, Haim seems to have joined forces with another of Leon's Salonica-friends-now-living-in-Marseille, Nissim Mizrachi, whose letters to Leon position him as a key figure in the Young Salonica Gang in Marseille. Quite a few letters that Leon received from them during the year show that on top of the mutual endeavour to make good in the new country, they maintained a strong and animated friendship. All were still young, single men at the time, so often, the letters are strewn with hints that they dealt not only in commerce.

Leon's relationship with each of his friends portrays quite a complex and varied social network. Nissim Mizrachi, perhaps the most dominant of the lot, gives his address and title as Courtier Representant, Café & Autres Denrées Coloniales, 52 rue du Coq, Marseille, seems to be in some connection as a broker with Salem & Amar, and is quite a lively, even outrageous correspondent. As is clear from the rowdy tone of the first of the 1926 letters written on January 26th, his friendship with Leon preceded their business association. If the proverb "tell me who your friends are and I will tell you who you are", is of any use, Leon's character is illuminated in quite an unexpected light.

Dear Leon,

… Long time…I hope you still remember me…you stopped writing, you monkey you, what are you doing in Paris? Have you fallen in love and forgotten about your friends? Write to me quickly, my dear Leon, because I do not know why I deserve such a long silence.

Do you realise that for the last month and a half, I have lived as a married man? Do you understand? I met a very cute woman in Spain who was in transition and stayed at my boarding house, and wink wink, fell for me and then, despite Mrs. Fure's objection, came to live with me in my room, with all her suitcases, ass and neck…

You can imagine the fun I had in her arms. But everything must come to an end and last Saturday she moved to Saint Clair near Toulon. I was heartbroken. Henri took care of me and took me to a dance, where we happened to meet two beautiful, heaven-sent women…

The funny thing is that since then, the four of us have been meeting every day, and that Henri, the maniac, has already slept with one of them while I haven't done anything with the other….

You see how miserable your Nissim is… please pray for me that she opens her legs as quickly as possible, because what annoys me most is seeing Henri get it before me. Besides that, my darling, nothing special. Business is very quiet. Hard, belt-tightening times. Health is good.

Mrs. Fure has sold the pension and we have a new landlord, who has a very nice daughter. Perhaps we should reserve her for you? So, you understand you are very welcome here.

Nissim Mizrachi

In a second letter six months later, on July 15th, Nissim continues along a similar vein.

My dear Leon,

For the past 15 days I have been carrying your smutty letter in my pocket and I am really ashamed that I have not yet found the time to answer you. Thank you very much for thinking of me and writing to me, my dear Leon. You can imagine how much I enjoy reading your news.

Business in Salonica is getting worse. Cafes are closing down and nothing can be done. Romance is also not great recently, because I have no money to spend. What's on offer on 5 Pisenson Street has been quite good, but I cannot afford any.[17]

So, nothing good to report, old man. I am still unemployed, pretty depressing, our piggy Henri helped himself out 3 months ago, so I'm pretty much alone here. No young people around and I am quite bored, often thinking about my dear Leon whom I miss a little too much.

I did see Leon last night, he told me he wrote to you. He's an old sour cucumber and since working as a shoe-maker he's been annoying everyone.

Don't forget to write to me.

Yours always,
Nissim

P.S. I am not sure what is the date today but I think it's Monday and that's enough.

These letters from his friends, Nissim's being just the first example, paint an interesting picture. It is now easier to visualize Leon fitting in the convivial and gay atmosphere of Paris in the 1930s. A period that had been immortalized in so many works of art, literature, theatre and cinema. As in other post-World War I, European capital cities, Paris too enjoyed the fact that during the war, women took on more social responsibilities, which strengthened their public position. Once the war was over, many women retained their improved social status and refused to return to the old pre-war traditional gender roles. In terms of fashion, Art Deco became, by mid-decade, the governing fashion where the ideal new woman was a tomboy, young, slim, athletic, short-haired and short-skirted, almost androgynous in appearance; a friend and an equal rather than a passive dependent.

In addition, the presence of many American cultural figures such as the writers Djuna Barnes (1892–1982), Samuel Beckett (1906–1989), Kay Boyle (1902–1992), John Dos Passos (1896–1970), F. Scott Fitzgerald (1896–1940), Ford Madox Ford (1873–1939),Hilda Doolittle (1886–1961), Ernest Hemingway (1899–1961), Anaïs Nin (1903–1977), Ezra Pound (1885–1972) and Gertrude Stein (1874–1946) as well as artists such as Marcel Duchamp (1887–1968) and Henri Matisse (1869–1954), musicians such as Igor Stravinsky (1882–1971), created a very lively and experimental cultural scene that contributed to what was later termed the Roaring Twenties, giving birth to Dadaism, which to date has exerted a huge influence over the development of cultural perception around the world.

It must be remembered that the foreign influence on Parisian life was a result of the fact that the end of World War I brought a strengthening of the American dollar, which made Bohemian Paris very attractive to American citizens and whoever else had foreign income. You could live easily on a budget of a hundred dollars a month. For a few years, life in Paris was indeed painted by the attractive colours Nissim Mizrachi attributes to Leon's decision to stay in Paris.

Nissim mentions Leon's other Salonica friends, now living in Marseille, Leon Hasson, Haim and Albert S. Scialom. All three write to Leon during that year, showing an active and varied social network of emigrés. The lively letters share many intimate details, perhaps giving them all a sense of belonging, which they lack, being away from their hometown. Writing letters is an uncanny substitute for being at home. Leon's three friends in Marseille kept an even closer contact with one another, as they mention each other and common social activities in the letters. It is a fragmented picture, perhaps akin to a faded drawing found in a desk drawer. The reader needs to use imagination to conjure up the flesh and blood relationships that the letters testify to. Many details are missing, and the gaps are sometimes bigger than the actual data. Still, there is enough information, not least the emotional tone of the letters, to tell the story of their friendship.

The second of the Marseille bunch, after Nissim Mizrachi, is Leon Hasson, a shoemaker. In his three letters of that year, in March, July and October, he writes movingly and daringly about his dire employment and romantic situation, presumably responding to Leon's reports of a similar difficult situation, after he had broken loose from both Salem & Amar in Marseille and his brother, Isaac, in Paris. It is not hard to imagine the letters that Leon wrote that merited such a response from Hasson when he wrote in March:

My dear Leon,

... I see that in Paris, like in Marseille and other places, business is not bright. For the past two months, I have been short of orders for shoes, and in order to not lose all of my investment, my lawyer has recommended that I close the business for a while and try and work elsewhere. It is true that people will always need shoes, but at the moment, the cost of making them is too high.

Life in Marseille is becoming more and more expensive. If in the past you could live on 900 francs a month, today you need at least 1200 francs.

If you ever decide to come to Marseille, let me know. I think I can get you a temporary work on a regular basis. As the Arabs say: "Allah is great and everything works out as long as there is health".

Nissim is a pig. I hardly see him. If he writes to you, give him my regards... What can I tell you, my dear Leon? I hope that when the summer comes, I will get a chance for some proper holiday in the village.

So, keep writing,
L. Hasson

The second letter in July, again placing Nissim Mizrachi as the pivot of the group, shows that some progress has been made, or is expected to be made, regarding employment, allowing Hasson to think about settling down and getting married.

My dear Leon,

Judging by Mizrachi's letter, it seems you have a very low opinion of my friendship...You are wrong dear, and please do not confuse silence with forgetfulness. This idiot Mizrachi is here to testify that I keep asking about you. He has been sending your regards so I am glad you didn't forget me. Ok, and now for really important issues.

Do you know any Jewish girls whom I might like? I'm really bored with the ones I know. I'm 31 and have all my teeth... I am healthy in body and mind and I really want to get married. I could do with a nice dowry, anything in the region of 200,000 francs will be very welcome with the beautiful bride you will find for me.

This is a serious proposition. As I said before, get me a bride and I can guarantee you a job as an accountant. I know someone like you who earns a salary of 24,000 francs a year, plus percentages. Don't think I'm kidding you. It will be extra pleasure to have you as my accountant after I can be married to the lovely woman you will find for me. I trust you on this.

Since I started working again in sales and left the shoe-making operation, I see little of Nissim. If you were here, I'm sure our common boredom would have turned into happiness.

So, what are you up to? Are you also getting getting bored in Paris, a paradise for passion and life? Aren't you going to get married? Apart from the bright sun, Marseille is no joy for people like me who work non-stop. Except for the odd night out and an occasional museum visit, I am dead bored.

*Please write soon. Your letters are always a joy for me, even if I
don't write back as often as I should.*

L. Hasson

During the same month of October, Leon receives a job proposition from
another of his Marseille friends, Albert S. Scialom, showing that the option
of moving south has not been taken off the table.

My dear Leon,

*... Nissim told me that you miss Marseille and since you have a
good memory of La Canebière, you would like to come back.
I am looking for someone as good as you and I can offer you a job,
paying 900 francs a month and a small percentage of profits.*

*I intend to start an export agency and could use you to manage
it. You will get administrative and managerial assistance from a
friend of mine who is folding up his own firm. If you accept, this
might mean a very good financial opportunity.*

I am waiting for your reply and hope it will be positive.

Sincerely,
Albert

And as if such an offer was not a strong enough incentive, a few days later
in October, Leon received a letter from Nissim, delivering some urgent news
but also reinforcing Albert's offer.

My dear Leon,

*You must have received by now the sealed envelope sent to you
from the tax authorities. I am forewarning you, as I know you have
unfinished business there, and I took the precaution of writing
back to them saying your current address is unknown. This will
give you some time to sort it out.*

*Yesterday another notice arrived of your tax debts - 3340 francs.
I thought it would be best to inform Amar & Salem, which I did
this morning. So now Richard Salem has the notice and I hope he
deals with it on your behalf urgently.*

*I think it is best, my dear Leon, that you write directly to the
auditor at Rue Saint-Jacques explaining your situation and asking
him to send all letters related to your former business to Amar &
Salem at Garibaldi Boulevard and explain that they are the only
address for all issues regarding that shop.*

Ok, enough of that. And now for something better, I hope... you never stop writing how much you miss Marseille and La Canebière, and since I want you to be happy, I've been following a business opportunity for you here. Albert S. Scialom is in contact with many potential customers for his export agency and needs someone like you to help him. He therefore asked me to write to you. Also bear in mind that the Mizrachi & Levi firm are moving to Salonica so all their business will be passed on to Scialom!

I don't think the beginning will be easy but I also know of a possible partner whom you don't know who has moved to Marseille and who is willing to put in a lot of money if the business works well. Be assured Leon dear that this can be a great plan for you, at least in my opinion, much better than your current situation in Paris. Because with the 900 francs Albert is prepared to pay you, you can get by brilliantly here....

So, write me just a quick word to tell me if this interests you. Let me just remind you one last time that your Nissim loves you very much and hopes for only one thing, that one day he will join forces with his Leon, whom he loves the best.

Nissim

Leon's reply to Amar & Salem is another rare glimpse into his mind. He did not take long before he responded to the new development that Nissim wrote to him about. And he kept a typed carbon copy... While it is a formal letter, showing some degree of concern, Leon does not neglect to insert a personal note so as to maintain the friendly connection they have just salvaged after the Isaac episode.

Dear Sirs,

Mr. Mizrachi informs me that a 3340 francs tax notice for the store on Garibaldi Avenue has arrived and that he has given it to you. I hope you did what you needed to right away. I ask that you write to the auditor to send all further notices directly to you and tell them that you now run the company. I know that you want to get things straight with the authorities, like me. I would not want them to come breathing down my neck now that I am working, and take my money.

I want to ask you to explain to me the legal measures you took to close the shop. You can understand why I need that information.

I hope that all is well with you. I enjoy life in Paris which I like very much.

Best regards,
Leon Cohen

Two more letters from this period allow us a glimpse into Leon's mind. The first is a long and detailed letter to Nissim, where he explains why he cannot accept Albert's offer at that time. The second shorter letter, not quoted here as it basically repeats in a concise form what he wrote to Nissim, is to Albert himself where, while turning down his offer, he leaves the door slightly open to future collaboration. It is clear from both letters that he would rather be in Marseille but holds back for two reasons.

My dear Nissim,

Sorry for taking so long. It is because of laziness but also because of my health.

I was recently down with a strong case of flu and not far from bronchitis. I still have a strong cough. But I take care of myself and am improving. I will have to be very careful all winter, because the weather in Paris can change and it is best not to be surprised by it.

I read your letter carefully and I thank you very much for your friendship. The opportunity you found for me in Marseille is very interesting and I've been thinking about it a lot during all this time. I say "I thought" a lot because if I had only myself to think about, I would have decided right away. I could live anywhere, if I could rely on a steady income and just think of myself. But you know my situation and I can't think of myself alone. For many reasons, many of which are unrelated to my wishes, if I stay in France, I must stay in Paris and not in Marseille. It will take me a very long time explaining all the reasons why I have to make this decision. But you can understand that if my parents were to come to France, it's better for them to be near my brother and be based in Paris. Today, I can earn about 1500 francs a month in Paris and I am sure I can earn more in the future. The salary that Albert Scialom offers is less than that, so moving to Marseille would not improve my position.

Still, as I told you, personally I would rather be in Marseille than in Paris. I have faith in Albert's abilities and if he does succeed, we can talk later to see how we can collaborate. I am sure he will need an active and dedicated partner, and I would love to work with him. We'll just have to wait to see if he can offer me a better wage.

Please share this letter with Albert and assure him that I would be very happy to start working for him if his business fulfils my reasonable needs. I think that I can complement him very well and together develop a great business in Marseille and France. This could be very successful if we work on it smartly and with energy.

Please convey all this to Albert and keep me informed of his plans.
Lots of love,
Leon

Considering the economic situation in Salonica during those years, it is not hard to understand why Leon was so determined to move his family away from Greece. As the historian Steven Bauman writes, the economic difficulties that affected the Jewish community in the city caused those who could to leave and seek their fortunes elsewhere. As a result of the influx of new populations into the city after the Second Balkan War, the Jewish community found itself in greater difficulty. The declining population that remained in Salonica suffered the loss of those who left.[18]

The year is drawing to a close, and in November, Benico Segura, Leon's old friend and a close and dedicated friend of the Cohens in Salonica, writes a revealing letter, updating Leon and encouraging him.

My dear Leon,

Your postcard from the 11th found us alive, which means we are not yet dead... Therefore you will have the honour to receive an answer from us, despite a slight delay.

I never claimed to be regular in my correspondence. I've always warned you about my laziness and inattention, so you can't expect many letters from me. But our true friendship should not suffer and I have no doubt that you will be content with my few lines. The main thing is to remind me to do this from time to time. But let's move on to more important things.

About two weeks ago, I went to visit your mother. She was of course glad to see me. Apparently, she sees a resemblance between us... I don't think you're as ugly as me and hope that the City of Lights hasn't changed you for the worse. But let's get back to the topic of your mother. During the whole time of the visit, she never stopped talking about you. That was the only topic we talked about. Your mother told me you are getting ready to move the whole family to Paris. I mainly wanted to see in this a confirmation of your decision to not move back to Greece, as many of your family members pressed upon you to do.

In my opinion, first of all, you do not have enough available funds to take care of the whole Cohen family in Paris. I'm not your mother. I am just an honest friend. That is why I want to understand what you intend to do with your family. Do you really want to bring everyone over? I think you should first start by bringing Benjamin to France. Find him some kind of work so that each month you can use your free cash to support the whole family.

I don't want to be negative about your brother, Isaac. I'm sure he promised your mother a decent amount of money if she came to live in Paris. I don't trust him to be able to fulfil such an obligation.

Under these conditions you should think first and only then act. If you are not sure you will be able to support the whole family in Paris, then you should move back to Salonica and at least make your mom happy, just by your presence.

Sorry if I'm getting too involved in family affairs, but I do this because of our deep and true friendship.

... life in Salonica is a little less monotonous than before. There is more traffic on the streets, more activity...Business? Mmm... Not brilliant. The crisis, the famous crisis, is going to be a disease that we keep hoping to overcome but cannot. I think it is probably the same everywhere, more or less.

Best of love,
Benico

P.S.: My brother seems to be over-doing it with his orders. I really regret giving him your address. If he happens to carry on like this, write to him and tell him in a nice way that you can't handle his orders because you are too busy. As a compensation, I gave your family free tickets to the Cinema of the Tour Blanche. Don't thank me. I do it happily.

Benico

Thus, 1926 drew to an end. It was a turbulent year for Leon. It began with hopes of a joint business venture with Isaac, which seemed to have petered out almost as fast as it was conceived, leaving perhaps hard feelings between the two. It certainly caused a lot of practical difficulties for Leon, which he seemed to have been able to overcome, both in the sense of his work and his ambition to better the fate of his family in Salonica. It was that, after all, which motivated him in the first place to leave Salonica and move to France.

Leon was still unsure as to his permanent base in France, being drawn to Marseille where several of his Salonica friends had moved to during the year. The temptation was great, but he resisted it. He had a plan. After recovering from the drawback with Isaac, which nearly sent him back to Salonica, defeated, he decided that his goal was to bring over the rest of his family from Greece, where the political and economic situation was not improving for the Greek people in general and the Jewish community in particular, having Theodoros Pangalos (1878–1952) as a dictator for most of the year. Combined with the beginning of Francisco Franco's (1892–1975) rule in Spain and the continuing rule of Benito Mussolini in Italy, Europe was not a particularly optimistic place as far as human rights and freedom were concerned.

1927 – Searching for the lost home

The Salonica Cohen family was all but annihilated by the Nazi occupation of Greece and France and the collaboration with the local police and civilian forces.

Seventy years on, I struggle to tell myself that there is no real need to continue exploring the painful past. There is no actual need to piece together the life of Leon Cohen from the letters, cards, photos and scraps of paper that were found. It will not bring him back to life (Figure 16).

Writing this, I know that it is futile to try and stop delving into the gaping hole of piecing together the torn bits of fabric that form the Cohen testimony. Stopping would amount to an abandonment of the memory. That cannot be done. Even though it is a dark and depressing endeavour, it needs to be kept at, knowing that it can never end; it can never reach a conclusion. The outcome is known at the beginning. There is no point in doing it apart from the endeavour itself. It leads nowhere but back onto itself. Remembering for remembrance's sake. There is no added value. No lesson can be learnt. It is futile and yet inevitable.

One flicker of light does appear in what appears to be a closed circuit of remembering: the new connections made with the relatives found in France. The discovery of the family of Bondy Saül, Leon's wife, opened new horizons (Figure 17). Apart from the fact that it was there, in their Provence home, that three boxes of letters were kept and then found, thus allowing the painful, futile and inevitable delving into the past, it is equally significant that new familial connections were made.

First, with Mireille Florent Saül, Bondy's niece who was two years old when her aunt, uncle and cousins were taken from their Rue Le Goff apartment to Drancy and then to their deaths in Auschwitz. Then the connection with her daughter, Marianne Leloir. Even though the relation is not based

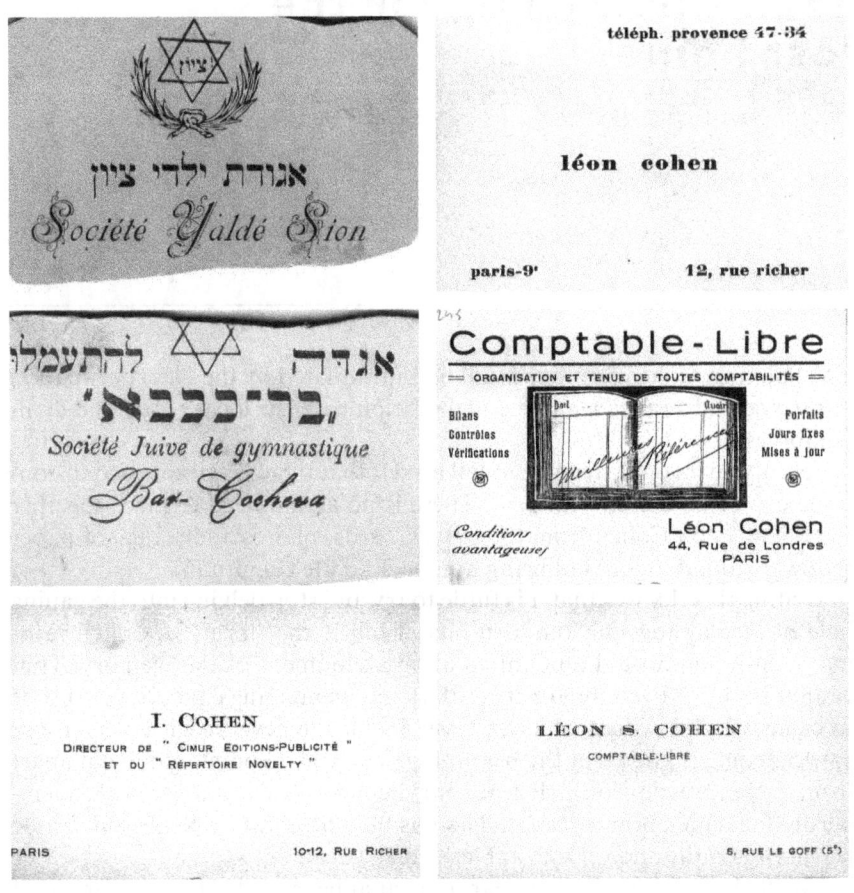

Figure 16 Leon Cohen's Cards.

upon blood ties, it is the only connection left available to try and piece together the coherency that was the Cohen family, a coherency eradicated, almost completely, by the Nazis and their allies.

If the translating, deciphering and piecing together of the Cohen letters is a form of monument, the connection with the Saül/Florent/Leloir family is a key to a young sapling growing in the present, taking in oxygen and exhuming life and hope for the future.

Back to the past. It is still 1927. The year opened with Leon subscribing to a sports club: Club Athlétique des Sports Généraux (CASG) on 112 Avenue Kléber. CASG was established in 1903 as the sports club of the bank "Société Générale". The club had a football team that played in the Parisian

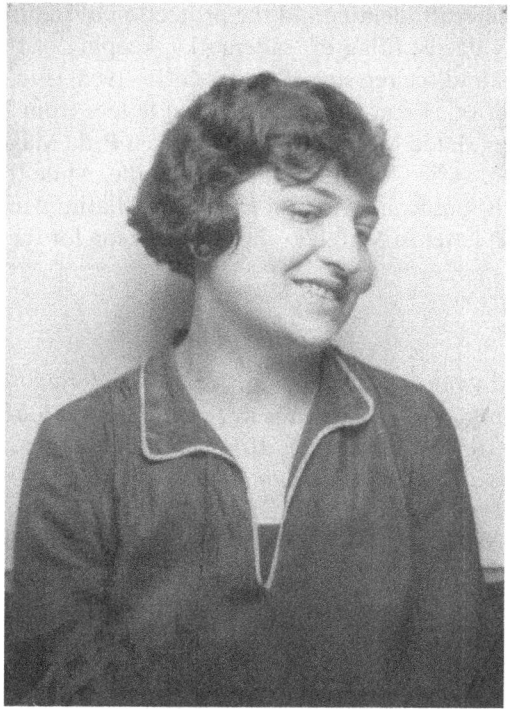

Figure 17 Bondy Cohen.

league and reached its peak between 1915 and 1925 when it won several local cups. It was still active until 1951. Today, the building is the location of the famous Centre d'Affaires Paris Trocadéro. Presumably, Leon registered in the club as a fan of the football team, which gave its best performance during these years. So, Leon was a football fan! What matches did he go to?

Having apparently given up his idea of moving back to Salonica, Leon was still entangled with affairs in Marseille. A tax demand popped up in March, job offers were circulated by his friends in Marseille and he seemed himself to be still considering a move down south. He also changed his address again. He left 96 rue Doudeauville sometime during the year and took up residence in Hotel Atlantic at 44 rue de Londres, a hotel still operating today.

In August of the same year, he is registered with the Tribunal de commerce de la Seine. Established in 1790, the commercial court was composed of elected judges who settled disputes between traders or associates of commercial companies that examined disputes over commercial acts and settled bankruptcies and liquidations. In addition, the registry of the commercial court assumed important administrative responsibilities in terms of trade and craft identity and the protection of industrial property: filing of company deeds, filing of trademarks, keeping of the commercial register from 1919 and the register of trades (1936–1962) (Figure 18).

During that period, Leon also received two letters from Nissim Mizrachi. The first letter, dated March 18th, is sent from P. de Mayo, Bonneterie-Confection-Tissue, at 53 Cours Belsunce, Marseille, while the second one, dated June 28th, is sent from Misrachi Frères, at Allatini 9 in Salonica. The content of the first letter in March explains the reason for the move.

Dear Leon,

... I can imagine your face when you receive this letter because you probably think your Nissim doesn't remember you because I haven't written to you in so long. Don't think like that. Your Nissim continues to think of his dumb Leon, but because of the circumstances, I couldn't write to you. If I told you everything that had happened lately... In January, I had a few polyps removed from

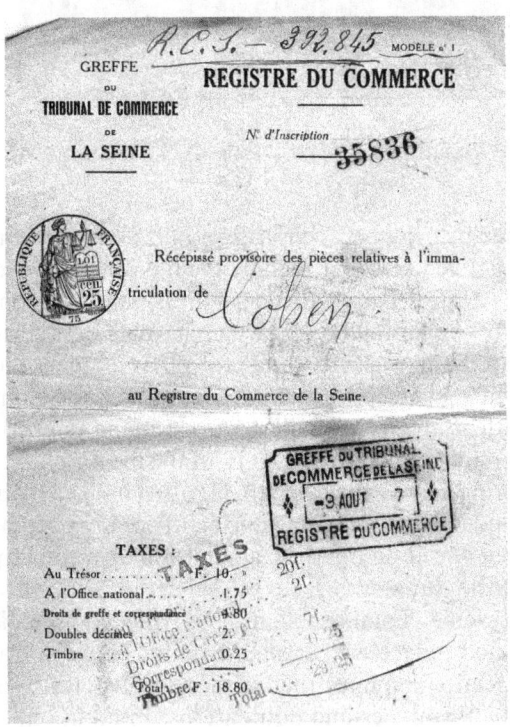

Figure 18 Tribunal de commerce de la Seine.

*my throat. They were quite painful over time. I spent two weeks
in hospital. In February, I felt better but there was a messy story
with … (Unclear). So it was all too much for me, dear Leon, that I
decided to go back to Salonica and work with my brothers.*

*I imagine you are now wondering why this stupid Nissim confuses
your mind with all these stories. So, here it is. This morning as
I was leaving my house, my landlord gave me this notice that
I am attaching here which shows that Amar & Salem have not
yet finished their business with the tax authority regarding the
business related to you. I immediately approached Mr. Balsha, the
new owner of your previous business, and asked for explanations.
He answered me pleasantly that he was willing to pay up what was
due on his account.*

*I then visited Amar & Salem and talked with Richard. Nothing
came out of our conversation, as usual. All the letters he received
were sent back with "address unknown" written on them. He asked
me to do exactly the same with the letter I received and even asked
me not to tell you anything. You know, my dear Leonico, that I
will do you no harm, so I told him I couldn't do what he asked me
to do and I would let you know right away so you could take care
of it. Either you start saving up now so that one day you can pay
the taxes, or if you do nothing, find someone to handle it on your
behalf. Richard dared to say that if you are going to trouble them,
they will go to your new bosses to take money out of your salary
until they get back the 3000 francs you allegedly owe them…*

Nissim

Leon responded almost immediately in a letter dated March 21st addressed to S.M. Franses in Marseille, for whom he had worked before.

Mr. Franses,

*I am sorry to take advantage of your trip to Marseille to request
that you contact your nephew Richard about a very serious issue
for me. When I worked for him, they listed a small grocery shop
with almost no income in my name, which, because it didn't work
well, was sold later. Because I am in Paris, I have given Richard
a power of attorney to handle the sale of the shop, to ensure that
I will be completely free from this business. Some time ago, I
got a tax demand from the government regarding this shop. I
immediately asked Richard to do as we agreed, and pay them and
write to the auditor at Rue Saint-Jacques to inform them of the
change in the ownership.*

Today a friend of mine from Marseille wrote that the tax authority has written and threatened consequences unless I pay them 3915 francs. Amar & Salem pretend not to know anything about this, which is very surprising, as I have always been a very dedicated and serious worker for them. Richard should know that there is no way to avoid the tax authority. And since he did not finalize the sale as we agreed, he has to pay the amount required by the tax authority. Even before the sale, they kept the business in my name to save themselves 3000–4000 francs.

It seems to me that it is high time to pay this debt to the tax authority and relieve me of this business, as I have been asking for so long.

So I ask you to explain to Mr. Salem and Mr. Amar the grief that this is causing me. The tax authorities will soon find my address in Paris and I will then have to come to Marseille myself and explain what happened. Sooner or later, they will have to pay. If they have anything else to ask of me, I'm still here to be accountable. I'm not a thief. If I had 4000 francs, I would have paid long ago and then claimed the money from Richard. But I know my rights. I don't have that amount and because I'm a foreigner, I might be expelled from the country. I believe that Richard would not want that hanging over his head.

Once again, Mr. Frances, I apologize for involving you and I trust you to explain the matter to Richard so that he will get it fixed.

Regards,
Leon

Next, Leon hears from Nissim Mizrachi, who had already returned to Salonica as he had promised. On June 28th, he writes.

My dear Leon,

I know you must be mad with me for not writing for so long.

I see your brothers often and they keep me informed about you. I met Henri last week and he told me he received a letter from you stating that you intend to leave your job at Fils Frances and look for something better somewhere.

As expected, your mom is a little worried about you and to calm her down, I went to visit her last Saturday, we spent a lot of time together and talked about you all the time. From what

I understand, you don't feel so great, so my dear Leon, be strong, don't worry. No one in this world dies of starvation. Even if you do not find work immediately, do not lose hope for a moment.

I would very much like, my dear Leon, to hear your news directly. What do you plan to do? Do you want to start your own business? If you need a partner to help you with revenue, tell me. I am at your disposal.

For me, life here is harder than we wish to believe. I haven't closed any firm deals as yet, but I did manage to make some coffee trade deals with Marseille, and still think I'll be able to set up my store soon.

Nissim

Several letters during July indicate how busy Leon was still trying to plan a move back to Marseille. On July 12th, he received a letter from a place he had hoped to use as lodging. It is the clearest evidence that he had indeed lived in Marseille when he first arrived in France, as he was seeking to lodge back with his old landlady, who this time had to turn him down, but in such a tone that indicated a warm and quite intimate acquaintance with him. It is indeed the only evidence I have so far that Leon had indeed first resided in Marseille.

Dear Sir,

I received your letter with many thanks. Sorry I didn't write you a New Year's letter. I lost your card and forgot to answer. I am now in a hurry to answer your question. I apologize but I no longer own a pension. The room where you lived no longer exists. I turned it into a living room and the other two rooms are already rented.

If you still intend to arrive in Marseille, you can write to me a few days before your arrival and I can find you a very nice room on République Blvd., which costs 160 francs and could suit you well. As for living expenses, I know men who spend 6.5 francs on a good meal, including wine.

I'm waiting for news from you.

Best, L. Huc

And then a couple of letters from Omry, a relative of David Salem and a friend of Nissim, responding to Leon's enquiries. The first letter is dated July 26th.

My dear Leon,

I got your letter of the 10th. I read it with much interest and my delay is only a sign of how busy I have been. David (Amar) is in the mountains with my sister and my mother has gone to Paris. I thought a lot about what you wrote. As you know, I've the highest regard for you. I know how honest and capable you are. I would love to help you. I had thought of trying to find you work as a broker or representative in Marseille, but after talking with many colleagues in the field, I don't think this is a good time for you to make such a move. You know how disappointed with brokership our Nissim (Mizrachi) was before he left Marseille.

Raphael Eryas is now focusing on the wool business in Constantinople. I would love to send you encouraging news and offer you something positive, dear Leon. I know very well how difficult the current period is, and that it is very difficult to get new things off the ground. Even so, dear Leon, you don't have to give up. I know how talented you are, and I am sure that before long you will succeed. Meanwhile, I will continue to look for something in Marseille.

I hope to be in Paris in about 15 days and to see you then. I remain your dedicated friend.

Omry

And then on August 11th.

My dear Leon,

... There is an interesting job available...Raphael Eryas, the wool merchant, has almost completely stopped trading coffee. While talking to him, the need to hire someone to help him came up and told him I could convince you to leave Paris if he could secure you an income in Marseille. After a good few days of deliberations, here's what I managed to come up with: 800 francs a month, and 15% share of profits. Eryas has promised me, and I think I believe him, that he earns 50,000 francs a year and that with your help, he hopes to increase that... He has found a place in the city which he will set up as an office. There will be a trial period of six months. If at the end of this period you are both happy with the arrangement, you can commit and sign a contract for 3 years.

Does that suit you? Write me or send me a telegram... There was another link I have tried to follow up for you in property evaluation but so far it has not materialised...

If I arrive in Paris around August 20th, I will write to you to make an appointment with you, unless you prefer to come here to Marseille straight away.

Waiting to hear from you.

Omry

There are only these two letters from Omry, both in 1927. It is clear from the nature of the letters that he was close with Leon and his family and so the fact that there are no more letters from him is yet another huge gap in the narrative. Presumably, he did not disappear from Leon's life but only stopped writing, or stopped writing such letters that Leon decided to keep. It has already been established that most of the correspondence that survived from these early years in France exhibited the kind of mixture of friends and business one would expect from a new immigrant trying to establish himself in the new country. Did Leon throw away other letters that he deemed at the time irrelevant? Or perhaps too personal? Was there a conscious mechanism at work, perhaps also motivated by the sense of threat he felt as an immigrant? As is clearly stated in his letter to M. Franses regarding the tax notice, he was well aware of his fragile status in France and perhaps only kept letters that could paint a positive picture of him? Naturally, in 1927, he could not have been aware of what was to happen, but perhaps the sense of alienation and threat was the unconscious force in his life. Was he already doomed to forever remain a stranger? Was he already suffering from *the secret wound*, a term I borrow from the work of French-Bulgarian psychoanalyst and philosopher Julia Kristeva (born 1941) on exile and strangeness?[19] Kristeva maintained that the individual's sense of belonging is never a solid, uniform verifiable entity, but rather an identity based upon a sense of *das unheimliche*, whereby what is familiar can become threatening at any time.

Was Leon indeed losing his contact with his mother and his home in Salonica? Despite the obvious sense of threat, and alongside the efforts of settling in France and deliberating where it would be best for him to establish himself, Salonica remained a live presence in Leon's life: not only through the reports by Nissim of his contact with his family but also through Benico, the same Benico who in 1926 managed to form a contact for Leon with his brother which offered him a ray of hope after the disappointment with Isaac. In 1927, only a single letter survived from him, written on an official headed paper of a company in Salonica called Publicitas Salonique, Agence Générale de Publicité at 7 rue Tsimisky in Salonica on September 24th. It is written with a hint of cynicism, indicating that Leon too was not always quick to reply, but still exhibiting a strong sense of comradeship that characterised the friendships Leon kept with his Salonica friends.

My dear Leon,

I wonder if it pleases you to receive my letters. I write again after you did not answer my last letter... I hope this letter makes you happy. As a reward you will get a little something from me...

I heard you are working in the advertising business in Paris. What a coincidence really: I've also been dealing with advertising for the last eight months and I'm pretty happy with it. It is a branch of great potential in Salonica. And because I'm pretty good at it, I hope to be good in this field. Already it has allowed me to break away from my brothers' firm after the argument I had with them.

I imagine that there is a lot of money to be made with all the advertising agencies. Salonica has only three agencies, so they all have a lot of work between them. Don't you want to come to work here? You've probably learned a lot there and you have a lot of experience and brilliant ideas. So along with your hard work, I'm sure that you can make a nice profit too. Maybe it's a weird idea to tell you to come and compete with me, but right now, I'm just thinking about the way companies are. And the truth is, I would love to see an old friend.

You wouldn't recognize your small hometown if one day you decide to come back. You will not believe what a drastic change has taken place, both in the city itself and in the way of life. You were born in a really amazing city and soon it will probably become the most beautiful in the Balkans. Not really boring here anymore. And take it from me as I was really bored here at first – it has become a vibrant, active city.

What's the news from Paris? I hope you don't get bored with it and that life isn't hard. I haven't seen your family in a while and they're probably mad at me for it.

Isaac and Nissim have dropped in to say hello and send their regards. They will write you separately. Isaac works in a wine and alcohol store that also produces Eau de Cologne. He runs a department there. Nissim has been working for some time as an accountant in a broker agency. He earns 2500 drachmas a month. As you can see, we are pretty happy with where we are. Health is fine and we hope you are well too.

Please write back soon with many details and dedicate as many minutes to the letter as I have!

Benico

Is that all I will ever know of 1927 in Leon's life? Was he indeed torn between Paris, Marseille and Salonica as appears from the letters, or are they not a true representation of what went on in his life at the time?

What were his inner thoughts? It is hard for me not to think about him in terms of exile, longing for home, grappling with questions of belonging, identity and a need to make a home for himself. Is it possible to live in a town which is not in your homeland and not feel all that?

Can I imagine Leon as a figure of The Outsider, so often described in the literature of his time? For instance, did he wander the streets of Paris seized with the same awe and estrangement as described by Henri Barbusse (1873–1935), in his book *Under Fire*, which Colin Wilson (1931–2013), in his book *The Outsider*, uses as the prototype for the modern outsider? Was he too seized with a passion for a woman, for any woman, as a way of coping with his desire to feel at home?[20]

Wilson was born four years before Barbusse died while writing a biography of Stalin in Moscow where he moved from his native France, driven by his Communist aspirations. An associate of Romain Rolland (1866–1944), Barbusse was a man of his time. The passion he ascribes to, the search for the Woman, who will relieve him of his existential despair, is beyond time. Countless men over the centuries searched for such redemption. Falling in love can provide the solitary man with the temporary uplifting of the spirit, so often mistakenly thought of as a solution to insoluble personal despair.

The examples are almost endless. Ten years after Wilson wrote his book, the exiled Argentinian writer, Julio Cortázar (1914–1984), who had spent most of his adulthood in the very same Paris, published his masterpiece *Hopscotch* in 1966 that opens with the protagonist's search for a mysterious woman called La Maga. He recounts the usual places he would usually find her in, searching for her along the Rue de Seine to the arch leading into the Quai de Conti, where he might see her leaning against a doorway, the olive-ashen light that floats along the river as she crossed back and forth on the Pont des Arts, or leaning over the iron rail looking at the water. He emphasizes that they would never make arrangements to meet as they were both convinced that casual meetings are just the opposite and that people who make dates are the same kind who need lines on their writing paper or who always squeeze up from the bottom on a tube of toothpaste.[21]

Men who are in some kind of existential identity search are bountiful. And more often than not, their search goes through the pursuit of women. It is the stuff of many an excellent *Bildungsroman*. Searching for the Woman is, in fact, a search for themselves as they would like to see reflected in the other. Was Leon Cohen in the process of living such an existence in those early years in Paris? Judging from the letters of his friends that tell of their own pursuit of women in Salonica and Marseille, it is safe to assume that he indeed was. If he was to record his own experience in the field, what would that have been like?

1928 – Isaac Cohen

I was born on March 15th 1962.

Freud left Vienna on his way to London via Paris on March 15th 1938.

The deportation of the Jews of Salonica began on March 15th 1943.

March 15th is also known as the Ides of March, the date on which Julius Caesar was assassinated in 44 BC.

In 1928, Martin Heidegger (1889–1976), the German existentialist philosopher, moved back to Freiburg, having spent four years in the dreary Marburg where he taught and had an affair with Hannah Arendt (1906–1975), the Jewish German-American philosopher.[22] Heidegger, who influenced Western philosophy more than any other intellectual except Freud, implicitly and explicitly supported the Nazi ideology, stayed in his cosy university post in Europe throughout the war and yet is still as influential as ever. While Arendt, who fled the Nazis to the USA as the war broke, exerted no less influence through her studies of tyranny and politics, exemplified in her controversial account of the Eichmann trial in Jerusalem in 1961.

Trying to make sense of the links between these dates and figures swirling in my mind, assuming that there is such a sense, consumes me. It is like walking through a labyrinth built on the edge of a cliff. Every now and then, it feels like I am losing track of my mission. What is my mission? What prize awaits me? The strangeness it evokes, the sense of alienation, is indeed Heideggerian, forcing me to contemplate again and again the *Dasein* of what I am trying to achieve.[23]

What I want to write remains unwritable. There isn't even such a word in English. The automatic Microsoft speller places a red, wavy line under that word, warning me that I am using a combination of letters that are unintelligible. I like that. That begins to approximate to what I am trying to do.

My grandmother Rita died when I was twenty-four years old and living in another country. I last saw her when I left Israel in 1983 when I was twenty-one years old.

The decision to return to Israel was not something that happened suddenly, one clear morning. It was not an event I can trace to a particular moment in time, a Tuesday afternoon. It was more like a limb that was always there, taken for granted, something that was a part of me since day 1, only that mostly it was just ignored, not needed in particular. It was only when it began to ache that it became noticeable. It needed attention.

The idea to return overland somehow made it easier. I thought that the journey should be prolonged, allow all my bits to rearrange and reassemble themselves before arriving back. Obviously, it was a delaying tactic. As if there was something else to be done first. I did not know what it was. At the end of the day, I booked a flight to Berlin. From Berlin, I had planned to make my way overland, by any means possible; train, car, boat and even foot, if necessary.

Before setting off, I looked at the map. Greece would be the last stop before leaving Europe and crossing the Mediterranean Sea to the other side. The first name that caught my eye on the map of Greece was Thessaloniki, or as I knew it – Salonica.

It was like finding something you did not realise you had lost. Salonica – of course, I will stop there on my way home. Salonica – the home of my maternal grandmother. At first, I only remembered little shreds of what later would become the monumental postmemory that filled my mind. But the vagueness of the cognitive trace was overwhelmed by an emotional tide that I then still could not understand. I just knew that I had to stop there. Stop and search. I did not yet know whom I was supposed to search for and it was only after a week when I spoke to my mother on the phone that the details began flooding in. I asked my mother to look at the letters Savta (grandmother) kept in the box. *Maybe the envelopes are still there too and you can look for the addresses.* I didn't know if they survived all the floods. The box hasn't been opened since she died.

The year was 1993. It took me six months to get from Berlin to Salonica. It would take me longer to recount why it took me so long. Most of it, I just don't remember. No notes were kept. I can trace the route – Berlin, Terezin, Auschwitz, Krakow, Budapest, Bucharest, Macedonia, Salonica. 1,877 km. Driving today through on the A1, it could take up to nineteen hours. No stop. By train, with minor stops and quite a few changes, about thirty-four hours. In effect, it took me three months before I reached Salonica. What happened along the way could be the subject for another book. In Salonica, I looked up the addresses that my mother had found for me, only to discover, unsurprisingly, that none of the original houses were still there. All destroyed since and rebuilt. I visited the Jewish Community Centre on Yom Kippur Eve, had a quick look through the local directory and even found someone bearing the name Parenti. He even looked like he could have been a family member. But my awareness was not yet aroused enough. The post-memory was still lurking, buried. I left Salonica in a hurry, took a ferry to Crete and spent a few weeks on the beach before finally getting on a ferry that took me to Haifa.

Meanwhile, though, after I had asked my mother to look for the en-velopes and while I was on my journey, she had started to look into the treasure of that box, the first box of the Cohen letters. Thus began the process I had described earlier that had eventually led to the discovery of the other three boxes... the translations of the letters... the evocation of the postmemory....

What was Leon doing during 1928? There is very little evidence in the boxes. He was still thinking about Marseille. Two telegrams addressed to his old address at 96 rue Doudeauville testify to that, inviting him to come to Marseille with a promise that all travel expenses would be covered.

It appeared that Leon stayed. His brother Isaac, on the other hand, never stopped travelling, sending cryptic messages like this one.

> *It is paradise here. I need to come back but have no address to return to. If you meet him, say there is a letter from the concierge. If you want to meet with us you will find us at seven pm on the cafe terrace. Whoever arrives first, waits for the other. If anyone asks, I am not here and I ask you to close the blinds to make sure people do not suspect we are not here. We will try to leave town soon.*
>
> *Phil*

Where was he writing this letter? He seems to be both enjoying his stay and at the same time needing shelter, instructing Leon not to disclose his where-abouts. Is this his departure letter from Paris, beginning his odyssey across France? He signs the letter *Phil* as he would many other times, presuming trying to hide his identity in case the letter falls into the wrong hands. Be-tween 1925 and 1940, Isaac wrote numerous cards to Leon. His presence seems to fill Leon's correspondence mostly with requests from his family for news from him. Requests that remain unanswered. What did happen to him? Did he settle down somewhere in France and was taken like his brothers to a concentration camp in 1942? Or did he leave France altogether and perhaps even survived? It will remain a mystery. To date, no trace has been found, not through archival searches in France, Israel or Salonica. The only evidence of his actual presence in the years after he left Salonica are two photographs taken a few years later after Leon and Bondy were married, but before they had children, sometime between 1934 and 1935.

The two photos, taken in what appears to be rapid succession, show a group of five individuals walking down a street (Figure 19).

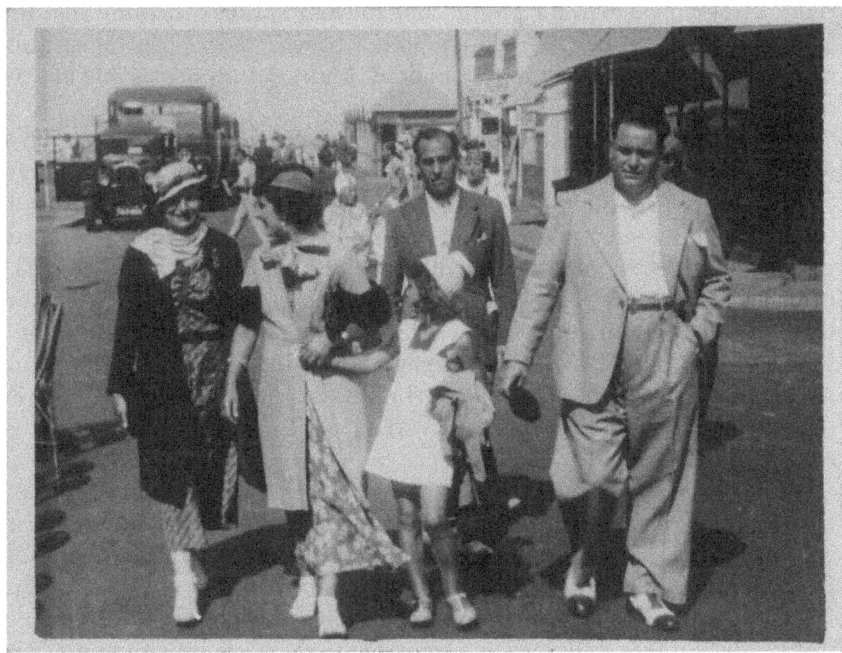

Figure 19 Leon, Bondy, Isaac and unknown figures.

Leon and Bondy are looking directly at the anonymous photographer. Isaac is walking beside them. Next to him is a woman who is turning her head towards Bondy and seems quite happy. And in between Isaac and that woman is a girl of about eight years old, holding the woman's hand and looking to her right. Isaac is holding *a yamuka* (a skull-cup) in his right hand, suggesting that they have all just been, or are on the way, to a synagogue or some other place where *a yamuka* is necessary. Holding the *yamuka* in his hand indicates that Isaac was not an observant Jew as such a person would not have taken it off his head unless, of course, he was wary lest he should be identified as a Jew and therefore concealing the fact.

It seems to be summer. They are lightly dressed, though still, the men wear jackets. The sun is in their eyes and they all squint. In the background, behind the group, some vehicles can be seen. Two of them are buses. In the centre of the picture, some people are seen wearing bathing costumes, in contrast to the elegant wear of the Cohens. In the farther background, there seem to be changing booths, indicating that this is somewhere near the beach. There is a photographer's shop on the far right, displaying a sign for photos and souvenirs, thus affirming that this is a place where tourists frequent, like a beach resort. The registration plates of the buses cannot be deciphered. Many details are visible but too obscure to make any sense.

Who are the woman and the child at the centre of the picture? Is it Martha, Isaac's Christian wife, next to him? And is the girl their daughter? A daughter nobody knew about and of whom there is absolutely no information in the correspondence or in the collective memory of future generations. The woman is wearing a wedding ring while Isaac wears a ring, but it is on his pinky finger. What does that mean? So, what were the Cohens doing in such festive dress walking along a promenade in a seaside resort in the middle of the summer on their way to a synagogue? As there are no Jewish holidays during the summer, is it safe to assume that they were attending someone's wedding, Bar-Mitzva or some other celebration?

Again, so little hard data upon which one can build mountains of speculations, leading in turn to wishful thinking regarding the fate of the people involved. There is no memory to substantiate any such speculation. But those speculations feed the ravenous creature that postmemory is. It is clear that Isaac was *the black sheep* of the family. It is an assertion that I was aware of from early childhood. Evidence supporting such a view is abundantly clear from the letters. He wrote very seldom to his family, and when he did, it was often to ask for assistance and money. Those requests were more demanding in nature than requests that would have solicited empathy and generosity from his family. It is hard to like the character of Isaac from the letters. Therefore, his image walking alongside Leon and Bondy with an unidentified woman and child gives rise to an abundant surge of irrational sense of hope that perhaps he did not fare as badly as it appeared. It is *Unheimliche* to think so but perhaps forgiven.

Back to the hard data. A dated card, March 14th, was sent by Isaac from Palais de la Bierre in 48 rue St-Jean, Nancy, perhaps a bar and a hotel, and today a branch of HSBC, the British multinational banking and financial services holding company. The need to hide is now accompanied by an explicit and detailed cry for help. Isaac is in some kind of trouble. And still, he invited Leon to come and join him in what he still describes as paradise.

Dear Leon,

I think you got my letters from yesterday. If not, please hurry and send me at least a thousand francs that I need right away. I also

*ask you to pay both bills which I enclose. If you don't have enough
money, just pay the first one. I apologize and hope you are not
angry. We are here from Sunday afternoon and in a few minutes we
leave again. I hope you have done everything necessary regarding
the bailiff. When you write, place your letter to me in a sealed
envelope, addressed to me, and place it in an envelope addressed to
the Casino manager.*

Kisses from Martha and Isaac

P.S.

*If you were here, you could live like kings. A full meal for 10
francs!*

A few months later, another card from the same place in Nancy dated
August 13th.

Dear Leon,

*Yesterday we arrived in Nancy. The route is very nice – good
air, but it rained all morning. There's not much to do here. All
businesses here have regular agents so we decided to return to Paris
via Reims, a well known place for champagne. I hope to succeed. I
need lots of money. Hope you get the cheque for a thousand francs.
Send it to me by mail to the address I gave you. We can only stay
one day in each city and therefore have to hurry. Sorry for all the
trouble but things need to get done. I hope you are well.*

Isaac

P.S.

*Instead of sending a telegram, please ring between two and three,
but not Tuesday. Hope the rain stops so we can go to Epinal, 60
miles from here.*

And then, as promised, a charming card from Epinal, 75 km south of
Nancy, sent the following day, August 14th, showing the view of the town.
But on the same day, a letter also arrives, written on the headed paper of
Grande Taverne, 26, Quai des Bons-Enfants, Epinal.

*Could not hear a thing on the awful phone. Still, it was very nice to hear
your voice from such a distance. We are having a good trip, even though
it is raining. I just realized Samuel didn't pay. You have to send us some*

money because we are desperate, right at the bottom. Tomorrow we will arrive at Gérardmer.

On Thursday, I will ring you again from between two and three o'clock. Try to be there.

The following day, August 16th, a card from Gérardmer, but now on a headed letter Casino Gérardmer, more information is given. The Casino was operated by E. Manouvrier and seems to be operating today at 3 Avenue de la ville de Vichy, 88400, located just by the lovely lac de Gérardmer.

Dear Leon,

Thanks for the money you sent. Arrived just in time because we were destitute. We arrived in the rain and storm yesterday and found out that there was a letter and a money transfer. You can imagine how pleased I was.... You do not know how grateful we both are. We shall stay here for a while, now that things are more settled, thanks to your kindness. I promise to make it up to you – we shall go the seaside in September.[24]

Isaac

Was the money needed for gambling in the casino? Even though he thanked Leon, the string of urgent and desperate postcards, letters and telegrams did not cease during August. Travelling around Gérardmer, Isaac sends out picture postcards from the Hohneck mountain, 20 km east to Gérardmer, the Col de la Schlucht, a mere 4 km north of the Hohneck mountain and then from yet another summit in the area, proudly stating that it was 1500 m high.

Once back in Casino Gérardmer, three letters are sent, all delivering the same desperate message – some money was received, but it is not enough. Isaac and Martha complain about the high cost of living and beg and plead with Leon to send them more money to allow them to be on their way. Isaac supplied Leon with minute detail as from whom he may be able to collect monies owed to him in Paris. Leon is fully engaged at this stage in running around and collecting Isaac's debts, but Isaac is never satisfied and in one letter after the other during the last week of August, sends Leon on what appears to be a wild goose chase.

Then, towards the end of August, Isaac and Martha are on the move again. They send a picture postcard from the Doller valley, 50 km east to Gérardmer. Then, another picture postcard from Colmar, 40 km north to Gérardmer. And then, on the 28th, they arrive at Hotel De Famille, Mulhouse, a further 60 km east of Gérardmer from which they send a letter on a headed letter carrying the name of the proprietor, G. Zumsteg-Schieb, carrying the same desperate pleas for money. The tone is both accusatory towards Leon for not responding fast enough and at the same time reconciliatory and apologetic for perhaps making him ill with all their requests.

The last message from Isaac in this string of communications is symbolic – a postcard from Belfort, 60 km southeast from Mulhouse, with the words: *Still waiting.*

All these picture postcards are addressed to Leon at 10 rue Richer, though he had not been living there for nearly three years. Does Isaac not know that? Is Leon hiding himself from his brother, or is it another evasive tactic by Isaac, now clearly trying to make his way down to the south?

1929 – The mystery woman

1929. A year with the least evidence to Leon's doings, apart from the last year, 1942.

A postcard from Isaac and Martha dated August 29th from Cap Gris-Nez in the north of France, showing that Isaac is again using the summertime to travel. This time, only a single card was preserved with nothing but the lovely view to suggest anything about his doings. We know he is still alive, still travelling. Does the fact that he does not ask for money signify anything? Perhaps, Leon did not keep the letters with the pleas for money that arrived during 1929. Perhaps, he only needed those of 1928 to remind him of what his brother was capable of. And perhaps, things were better for Isaac and Martha. One would like to believe that after the turmoil of the summer of 1928, he was able to take control of his life and settle himself.

The other letters of 1929 that Leon kept are the beginning of a correspondence that will go on for some years. The first three letters in the series introduce a woman of indeterminate age who seems to know Leon quite well, Jeanne Gilles.[25] What was the nature of their relationship?

Who was she, at 48 Rue de la Procession, Paris, a mere hour's walk from 44 rue de Londres where Leon was living at the time when she wrote those three letters in 1929? From future communication which went on until 1931, she seems to have been a former colleague of Leon's, perhaps a secretary or a typist, in a firm he had worked with. The first letter from her is dated March. Though addressing Leon in a formal way, suggesting indeed a former employer–employee relationship, there is an underlying, implicit and maybe even illicit, warmth, insinuating something else too...

... I will arrive quite late (3:30–4pm), on my way to measure a coat... Yesterday I saw Mr. Lesselier from Provence who said he has some business for you. Do you want to call him today? ... I ordered the stationery you asked me to. It will arrive around April 6th. I will check again in a few days to know the precise date.

See you later.

Jeanne

A second one from August

... I received your nice letter. Thanks. As your friend, let me tell you that you are really ridiculous for not coming to Celette. Life is here is so much cheaper and simpler. I know that you spend a lot of money in Paris. Is it because you have fallen in love? If it's anything else that prevented you from coming with me, then it is a great pity.

I will not be angry with you, but if possible, I would love to know what made you change your mind. I would have been very happy for you to be there. We could have fun. You would not have recognized me. I'm not who I used to be, I have learnt to have fun. We could have done so many things together.

When I went on vacation, I asked you what you were planning to do. You replied that you were travelling with your brother for 15 days. That's why I didn't offer you to come and have fun with me in Marseille, but that's what I wanted, you silly you! In 8 days I'll be back in the office, I'm not looking forward to all the work which is waiting for me!

What are you doing today? You may be bored. Serves you right! If you were here, you would be only having fun. With me as a friend. But now we are both sad, it's very sad, you know.

What a beautiful weather the last few days have been. I sunbathed a bit. You could have seen for yourself.

Goodbye Mr. Cohen, and if it pleases you, get on the train and spend as much time with me as you can, even just 4 or 5 days.

And the third from September

... I've got a couple of spare theatre tickets with me, if you fancy going. There's four of us (girls) going. I didn't see you in the morning. Did you fall asleep?

Unanswered questions. Scarcity of real data. The desire to know, to reconstruct and to form an image of the past all lead me to the realms of the imaginary. What I can't experience through actual evidence, I can imagine, make up. But is it allowed? Does it not offend Leon's memory? The idea that perhaps Jeanne somehow managed to survive the war and went on living, establishing a family and descendants who are still alive, is inevitable. There is no indication that she was Jewish, which increases the chances that she survived and was not amongst the six million Jews who died. But as it is known that overall twenty-five million people died as a direct result of the Nazi occupation of Europe, perhaps the chances seem slimmer.

I would like to think of her as the mystery woman in Leon's life. That would have added another dimension to the story. A love affair that led nowhere. A broken heart. Hers? His? The last relationship before Leon was to meet his wife Bondy several years later?

Let's say they worked in the same office. Leon was a free-lance account-ant, perhaps sharing secretarial assistance with another colleague who shared his office. His practice was good but modest. He could not afford a full-time secretary.

They put a small advert in the paper. They also asked around amongst their friends. It only took a few days before Jeanne responded. She first sent a letter of introduction, as was customary. They both liked her clear and ele-gant handwriting. They joked about what a woman with such a handwriting might look like. They had expectations.

When she entered their office for the appointment, they were not disap-pointed. There was something about the way she carried herself that left no doubt. The interview did not last for more than fifteen minutes. They hired her almost immediately, after they inquired for formal recommendations. Days later, when they all felt more at ease with one another, she teased them about that interview, commenting that she prepared for hours for an inter-view that last only fifteen minutes... if only she had known, she would not have bothered. Leon and his colleague felt a bit awkward at that, but her pearly, rolling laughter soon dissipated the tension.

Soon, they both had fantasies about her. Each tried to hide his attraction and treated her casually. It did not take long, though, before they confessed to each other, over a glass of pastis at the end of the day, that they were thinking of asking her out...

As I am writing this, I am becoming aware that I am in fact describing a tale which reminds me of the 1962 François Truffaut (1932–1984) film *Jules et Jim*. Starring Jeanne Moreau (1928–2017), it narrates a love triangle in-volving two men and a woman. Though based on a novel written in 1953 by Henri-Pierre Roché (1879–1959), its plot described French and Parisian life just after World War I. Roché was a figure in the Dada movement in Paris during the very same years that Leon was there, but he was lucky enough to move to New York where he spent the war years, only returning to France years after it was over.

I am awakened from this delirium with Moreau's voice in the opening scene of the film made in the year I was born. The screen remains dark for a short while, and a woman's voice can be heard as she says: *you said me: I love you. I said: wait. I was going to say: take me. You said to me: go away...* it was about 1912. Jules, a stranger to Paris...[26]

How I wish any of this were true. That Leon had had fierce love affairs with women like Catherine in the movie, a woman who would turn his life upside down and make him forget his loyalty to his closest friend. And then, he would come to his senses, realise his status as a stranger in the city, realize that she had been using him all along to fill that gaping hole in her, the hysteric yearning for a man she could despise. I can imagine Leon, over another glass of pastis at the end of a torturous weekend, confiding with his colleague that maybe they had made a mistake by hiring such an alluring secretary. Seeing the sadness in each other's eyes, they decide to let her go. With a downcast glance and a heavy and throbbing heart, they approach her with the news the following morning. Watching her storm out of the office leaving behind a scarf and a half-empty bottle of perfume they would then keep in the office's safe, they felt that they had let a fairy escape. But when the news of her engagement to an elderly Baron, residing in Aix-en-Provence, arrived a few months later, they could not tell the relief from the regret in their hearts. Alas!

1930 – Rita's wedding

As far as I know, Leon Cohen and Henry Miller never met. There is no evidence that they did. On the other hand, there is no evidence that they did not. What is clear is they both lived in Paris during the same period. Cohen was there from 1926 until his death in 1942. Miller first visited Paris in 1928, when he was thirty-seven years old, and then returned to live there in 1930 until 1940, when he returned to the USA having made a name for himself during that decade as the writer of *The Tropic of Cancer* and *The Tropic of Capricorn*, two books that were banned for years by the British and American establishment, since they contained what was then considered to be immoral and profane content, or in other words, slang, swear words and a lot of explicit and honest descriptions of sexual relationships. That kind of writing was confined in those days to the backrooms of society. It was only in 1961, thirty years later, that Miller's books were published in America. I would like to think, if my interpretation of Cohen's bachelorhood is not too fantastic, that he would have liked Miller's depictions of human lives.

Miller arrived in Paris, this time to stay, on March 4th 1930. He took up lodgings in a shabby hotel room on the Left Bank. He was dirt poor, having left the USA with only ten dollars in his pocket. He could not find a job as he didn't even have a *carte d'identité*. He was still recovering from the convoluted relationship he had with the woman he had left behind in the USA, who did not take long before re-appearing in his life, throwing him into more disarray. As she did not stay for too long, he was able to re-establish himself with help from his newly acquired friends and found himself staying in the living room of Richard Osborn, a banker friend from Connecticut, whom he got to know through his Austrian friend, Alfred Perlès. He was mainly reliant on the kindness of such acquaintances and luckily had his good wits with which he was able to charm enough people to be able to pull through each day.

His difficulties did not stop him from dedicating himself to doing what he had wanted to do in Paris, what had led him to leave his homeland – to write. Having tried to resurrect an old writing project and failed, he set to write what would later make him his name – *The Tropic of Cancer*. That book was in his eyes, the most honest approach, honesty even to the point of ugliness. While staying at Osborn's flat on Rue Auguste Bartholdi, he began writing it. It took him the best part of four years to complete. But it was only after he met Anaïs Nin in 1931 that he was really able to rise above the squalor of living in other people's living rooms and sleazy hotel rooms and enjoy the comforts of her patronage. With Perlès, he moved out of the shared room in Hotel Central at No.1 bis rue du Maine and moved to an apartment on the Avenue Anatole France in Clichy, where he developed the daily routine that gave birth to *The Tropic*. His description of that time is moving. He writes that the place he is living is at the Villa Borghese is clean, and there is not a crumb of dirt anywhere, but spiritually, he and his friends are all alone and dead. Having spent one year in Paris, he is still unsure what he was looking for there. He has no money and no hope, but still, he is the happiest man alive. He describes his surroundings in Montparnasse as predominately Jewish. It is an overwhelming presence for him, and still, he identifies with being Jewish, being ugly and self-hating.[27]

This was Miller's Paris in 1930. This was his view of Jews, already well-formed after he had spent his life in Brooklyn. Is this the worst of anti-Semitism Leon was experiencing in those years? Had he met Miller, what would he have said to him?

A major influence over Miller in Paris in those years was a Lithuanian Jew named Michael Fraenkel, whom he met at his studio at 18 rue Villa Seurat, where in later years, Lawrence Durrell would also stay with them. The themes of love and death were Fraenkel's as much as they were Miller's. The friendship between them was extremely important for Miller, but not only due to the inspiration he drew from him. He also hated him in a way that could suggest anti-Semitism but was mostly the self-hatred he seemed to marvel at. In a very few years, the context would change and what seem like literary and soul-searching reflections would turn into a very harsh reality. Miller himself stayed in Paris until July 14th 1939. Most of his friends had left, amongst them Durrell who went back to Corfu and Fraenkel who went to America. It was only then that he too boarded a boat in Marseille all the way to Corfu, where Durrell picked him up and brought him to his house at Kalami where he and his first wife, Nancy, were living.

And Leon Cohen? He was in Paris when Miller arrived and stayed after he had left, nine years later. During 1930, a photo survived showing him with a group of unidentified people. He seems to be at ease with them. They seemed to be lounging somewhere in a countryside setting. Do they look bohemian? Is it a justified interpretation to support my wishful thinking that perhaps he was also influenced by the like of Henry Miller? (Figure 20).

A single postcard sent by Isaac from Epinal October 27th, again sent to Leon's old address, this time to 96 rue Doudeauville, follows an unusually direct letter in October, showing that perhaps, it was not always Isaac who played rogue in their relationship.

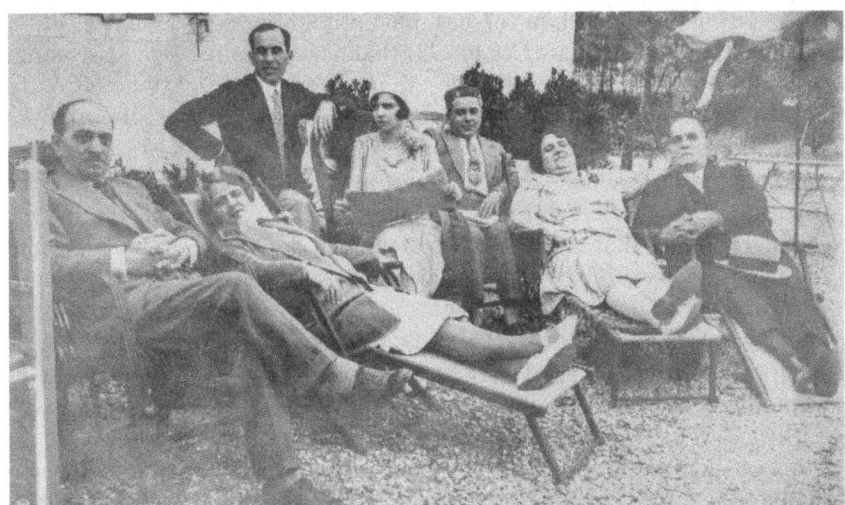

Figure 20 Leon Cohen and Friends circ. 1930.

Dear Leon,

I've been waiting all week to see you. I hope you're not upset.
Martha is annoyed. Sometimes you say things out of place. You
lose control because of your drinking. Have you heard anything
from Mom? Was she discharged from the hospital? I don't know
anything. But I assure you I very much want to get news from her.

Isaac

The mention of the family in Salonica in Isaac's letter shows that he was not indifferent to them, as he would be accused in later years. In this letter, it is Leon who appears in a different light. Has he changed? Has his behaviour become more unruly due to the affair he was perhaps still having with Jeanne? Or perhaps he did meet Henry Miller after all and was influenced by him…

Apart from the continuing and puzzling correspondence with Jeanne where it is still unclear how intimate their relationship was, the other significant item in the collection is the announcement of the engagement of Shmuel Parenti to Leon's younger sister, Rita, my grandmother.

Leon kept the newspaper clipping of the notice in the Axion newspaper, published in Salonica in Ladino on October 4th, which invited greeting visits on Saturday, October 4th [1930], 193 Migasso Alexandro Street.

The fact that Leon had kept that newspaper notice indicates how important the marriage was for him. It was a mutual sense of importance as Shmuel also kept the letter Leon sent him upon receiving the news (this letter first appears on p. 24). Not only did he keep it when he received it in Salonica in 1930, but also safeguarded it on the way to Palestine in 1934 and then through all the years, until the box of the letters was reopened in the 1990s.

It is not just a mere courtesy that Leon addressed the letter to Shmuel rather than to his sister. As Shmuel was a friend of his younger brother, Benjamin, who introduced the two to one another, it is highly likely that Leon too had met Shmuel before he left for Paris.

Dear Sam,

Allow me to address you in such an intimate way even before I can call you my dear brother-in-law? Is it necessary to greet you? Is it necessary to compliment you on your choice of a bride? I will only say that I wish you much happiness and a long life. I am beginning to grasp that that is true happiness: home, a loving, beautiful, clever, loyal and good-natured wife, one of us.

After one is married to such a woman, we can face life with more courage. I will be brief today and hope that you respond quickly so that we can get better acquainted. My brother Isaac also sends his greeting. He and his wife Martha are always busy. Even I only see him once or twice a week here in Paris and even that only briefly.

Leon

The actual circumstance of the very short engagement followed by the marriage of Shmuel Parenti and Rita Cohen is a story I became aware of from an early age. It was not an entirely happy story. Rita was two years older than Shmuel, and she was already twenty-eight years old, an age that in those years was considered quite advanced for a woman to remain single. At that time, Rita was already working as a teacher at the Alliance Israélite Universelle in Salonica where she had met a young colleague with whom she became intimate. It was a relationship that was not approved of by her family as he was not Jewish. She had to give it up and to accept the arranged marriage to Shmuel, her younger brother's friend and associate from the Theodore Herzl organization. She never spoke about that with me but confided this to her children. The identity of that other man in her life and the details of their relationship, like so many stories in this patched-up post-memory tale, were taken with her to her grave, leaving as wide a space for imagination as the reader chooses to take. I found myself often venturing into that space and filling it with my contributions, wondering whether it would have pleased her, the ultimate reader of this account. As that reading will not take place, it remains a troubling mystery.

1931 – Homesickness is not a disease, they said...

Perhaps, the most revealing letter of 1931, a year filled with economic distress, perhaps even of the whole collection, as it shows the depth of emotion and relationship maintained within the Paris–Salonica–Tel-Aviv triangle, is the letter Leon wrote on June 8th. Discovered in the box his sister Rita kept under her bed all the years since she arrived in Tel-Aviv three years later in 1934, it is a letter Leon addressed to his mother, Rachelle. Rita carried that letter with her, as she did with the letter sent to her husband-to-be. Little did she know that those letters would remain the only connections she would have with either Paris or Salonica to the end of her days in 1986. It is the clearest indication of how important Leon was for her. The letter was received when she was still in Salonica, already married to Shmuel and pregnant with her first daughter, Esther.

My dear mother,

I am very worried that I have had no news from home. What's going on?... I suppose this long silence stems from a bit of carelessness. However, if there was something wrong that happened, I would like to know the reason and no matter what. I'm waiting to hear from Benjamin, in response to the letters I sent him.

If I couldn't do anything for Rita's wedding, it's because I didn't have the means. I do everything possible to keep up here. And it's not always easy.

Don't forget that as long as I could, I did everything for the family. I'm not to blame if I can't do more...

Please send me news of what is happening to you through the letters of my brothers. Later when they realise it, they will know they should not leave a son without news of his mother, especially when the son is very far from home.

You may not be happy, but believe me, neither am I, and even less because of your unhappiness.

Hope to hear from you, my dear mother.

Kisses,
Leon

It is a letter that requires neither interpretation nor contextualization. Leon is homesick and begs his mother for comforting news. He is sad he missed the wedding of his sister and implicitly asks to be forgiven. He is aware of his mother's sadness and feels helpless. Above all, it is a testimony which Rita carried with her of their deep connection.

Alongside the sadness that the continuing exile caused Leon, the other evidence he had kept of 1931 was his developing relationship, still obscure in nature, with Jeanne. Several letters from her, now living in Neufchâtel, dating May–June, were kept in the boxes.[28] She was now living in a rather dull place, waiting for her marriage to take place. She writes to Leon in a very familiar manner. In the present string of letters, it is clear that she is helping Leon to establish himself as an accountant in Paris by typing out for him copies of a circular letter. She is also obviously very familiar with his family in Salonica. In one of the letters, dated May 11th 1931, she asks about his sister Rita and her planned wedding. It is clear that Leon had intended to return to Salonica for the wedding but could not. The disappointment he expressed in his letter to his mother is explained in the May letter from Jeanne.

Dear Mr Cohen

Your letter reached me this morning. Hopefully Mr Letellier's successive phone calls to reschedule your appointments are mere delays, for as I remember he always mentioned you in warm terms to Mr de B.. What's more, he seems to find you congenial. I am looking forward to you telling me how it turns out.

It's not a dishonour to be in need, though it is very much a nuisance, (as I, alas, know from experience). I suppose you are not living in luxury these days, as, what with the economic crisis dragging on, business is difficult. Don't you think it might be a good idea to look in other venues? This is what I suggest – send me the list of the firms where you would like to apply, and, following the example you will have drafted, I shall type out relevant letters. I still have my old typewriter, so it is all perfectly easy – do not even trouble yourself about paper, I have some.

Now, don't be "silly" and say "it's going to be a nuisance to her" or "it's going to add to her workload" – no, it will make her happy if, she is able to do you a tiny favour as a good friend. So do go ahead at once, you know I am offering quite willingly.

I am not surprised your stomach should have been upset, what with your most unwholesome diet, what you eat is appallingly unhealthy – too much meat, too few vegetables – if you had followed my girlish advice, you would have been the better for it... You make a joke of how your troubles would amuse me...

As for me, I have been laid up for ten days or so. I got frostbite on my heels, the right heel was close to ulceration. My ankles were terribly swollen, and my feet had a greenish tinge. The doctor claims it is due to very bad blood circulation. I am much better now but as the spot that was nearly ulcerated is still very painful, I am unable to bear the stiffness of a shoe.

I do not yet know when I shall return to Paris, I think that I should know quite soon whether I shall join my fiancé or that he returns here – but do rest assured I shall let you know, so we may have a few pleasant, friendly hours together.

If you were to move from your present hotel, do let me know, though it is true I have your brother's address so I could get the information from him if the occasion were to arise – are you back on friendly terms with him?

Best wishes – do hurry up and make that list.

Warmly yours, your good friend, Jeanne

A few months later on May 11th, she writes again.

Dear Mr Cohen

I am still waiting for your letter so that I can type out copies. Come on, admit it, you don't trust the sincerity of my offer, though, believe me, I would have been very happy to do you this small favour.

What are you up to these days? I don't know whether you are still at the office. Did Mr Letellier finally keep that appointment with you, and did you get that job?

My congratulations on the cards you made, they are very cleverly made.

Is your sister Rita married now? Have you been able to act on that nice plan of yours? You intentions are very good.

Are you in good health? Still nursing your stomach?

As for me, since I still have my resolutions, I have no reason to complain.

I was to join my fiancé in March, all that was missing was the permission of the firm where he is an employee – it was refused – fortunately my fiancé had set out his terms – either consent to my joining him or let him go back home, so he was allowed to come back. As a result, I think I should be able to leave Bourtais at the end of May and be back sometime in July. The present economic crisis has caused us to be separated for a long time. No need for me to spell out how glad I am at the prospect of seeing him again very soon. As soon as he is back we shall be married. We don't yet know where we shall live.

What about you, you fussy old bachelor, are you going to decide on marriage at last? It is high time, for I can tell you are going to become bald very quickly.

On Thursday I am to go to the Paramount-Opéra in Reims[29] *to see a performance of "The Round of Hours", you know André Barry is my favourite singer. Do you like "Dannie"? I heard it recently as a solo, I love his soothing and captivating voice.*

A very affectionate handshake from your former little colleague, Jeanne

And on June 8th

Dear Mr Cohen

I received your letter of the 6th yesterday – Sunday.

In two or three days I shall send you fifty letters following the example you suggested. Please tell me, quite sincerely and immediately, if it is enough – for I have no idea how many you need – do tell me exactly.

As for the envelopes, if you want them typed, you would need to give me lists, as unfortunately there is no phone book here in Neufchâtel!!! You forget we are out in the sticks![30] *I am enclosing an envelope of the type I can buy in Neufchâtel to use for my business letters – I think it is adequate and it is quite inexpensive. If I were to buy 500 or a thousand I would I think I would be given a discount, in fact I am sure I would.*

I am very happy to be able to do you this small favour. Believe me I am more than willing to do so, for the sake of our friendship.

A few days ago I got a telegram from my fiancé letting me know he would arrive in August, and yesterday I got a long letter giving me a few typing jobs.

His health is not good at all – he keeps having fits...

Your letter of the 17th and the cards did reach me. I had indeed presumed you were spending Whit Sunday holiday with your brother and sister-in-law.

The issue of L'Figure about the Colonial Exhibition was quite good. Needless to say I will and shall see it for myself some day and the article will be a good guide.

Yesterday I spent my day off at the dog exhibition in Reims. The weather was frightful. My six puppies are getting sweeter and sweeter. Every three hours I give them Quaker Oats milk porridge; they breast feed from their mother frequently, they do like their food! I am very fond of them and shall be very sad when my parents let them go at the end of the month.

Affectionately yours, Jeanne

Followed eight days later on June 9th

Dear Mr Cohen

I am enclosing 56 completed letters.

I was unable to type them out with black carbon paper as I unthinkingly went on using the "carbone violet noiseless spécial" out of habit.

There is no need for you to proof-read them, it has all been done and there are no typos.

I shall be looking forward to a note from you telling me whether it is enough, if not, please tell me how many you want. I am holding on to the example you sent.

How dreadful the weather is!

Jeanne
    Not a day passed and another letter on June 10th

Dear Mr Cohen

As it is ever my habit to speak my mind plainly, I shall say you expressed yourself like an imbecile...Have you actually gone soft in the head?

When you ask someone to "type out a few and date them so there are 10 to 15 a day", one naturally concludes you want rather more than twenty all in all.

Nor did you tell me you had had 1000 circular copies printed out!

Concerning the envelopes, I went to see the shopkeeper this morning. The owner was not present so I can't yet get a discount. So, even if I were to buy a thousand, it would amount to 28F which boils down to the same as the envelopes you will send from Paris, since the postage price would have to be added, and that would be relatively high. I placed an order with no obligation to buy if the arrangement does not seem suitable to you. However, since they only restock once a week, and that on Tuesdays, I shan't have them until next Tuesday. It's up to you. You can also compare the quality of my envelopes with what you can get in Paris at the same price, since it is impossible to find a white envelope of that kind for the same price from any stationers, even in Reims.

In the future you may find it useful to know that in a circular letter the right thing to do is to have the mention "date as postmarked" inserted where the date should be. It is much more accurate than choosing June the 5th and mail them out ten or 15 days later.

You may not have picked the best time to send these out, I'm afraid, as the summer holiday period is near, as you seem to forget.

Send me the addresses as soon as possible, and make a mark next to the names of the people I am to write to. There is no need to put your address on the other side of the envelope. I think it would waste too much time. If any letters should be undelivered they would be sent back to you.

I do hope the typed letters you send me are typed by you yourself – for I would hate for any person on the payroll of one of the firms you work for to know about your private business.

Please do drop me a line to confirm my order of the envelopes. My father-in-law is away today, I have not been able to ask him what might be the least expensive way to send you the said envelopes. I think it will be as "samples".

Please do tell me how many to send in each package. If you make yourself clear and accurate you will be quite satisfied with your typist-friend…

I am not writing more today as I want to complete a job for my fiancé so I am ready to start on yours as soon as I receive it.

Bother! It's only just now occurred to me – I have a purple ribbon, what colour did you choose? It is black? If such were the case, would you mind very much? Should I order a black ribbon? What a setback that would be! Especially as they take their time about it.

My apologies for this letter's rude beginning – please excuse it for the sake of my friendship, as expressed in my warm regards

PS

I passed on your regards to my mother and she sends hers.

Jeanne

What can one gather from the fact the Leon kept the correspondence with Jeanne all those years? It seems they met through work but with the years they developed their relationship beyond that. Was there ever a romantic aspect? If so, it is very gently insinuated, especially in the early letter from 1929.

One missing link follows the other. Isaac, whom Jeanne mentions in her letters, strengthening the assumption that her connection with the Cohens was more than casual, is still moving around France, he sends Leon messages, reports of his doings and cries for help.

On April 4th, a beautiful picture postcard from Le pont des Fées in Gérardmer, which today seems to have turned into a restaurant. It is correctly addressed to Leon's current address, 44 rue de Londres.

A week later, on April 11th, Isaac sends Leon to collect his mail. He writes on a business visiting card with an official title – Reportoire Novelty – Administration et publicité, 10–12 rue Richer. Further typed details on the cards describe the company as dealing with "Reportoires-programmes des concerts, des grand hôtels, cafés, brasseries et restaurants de luxe".

The following day, Isaac is back in Nancy. Writing from Hôtel du Palais which seems to be a different name to the place he stayed in a year before at 48 rue St-Jean, he writes:

Dear Leon,

... I've been trying to call you on the phone... We arrived at Nancy at 8 am, very tired. Please, help me and check every other day in the office and pick up the mail, because I'm afraid I'll get urgent blue papers (telegrams).

If there are any, open them, read what's important and try to get in touch with me in Nancy. I will stay here till Wednesday. Thursday I have to go to Lille. Tomorrow I will go to Epinal and on Friday to another town, Gerardmer. On Wednesday we will pass through Nancy and pick up the mail.

On Wednesday the 15th, my employee will transfer some money.
Please, be nice and check in the evening to take the money and all
unpaid bills.

Too bad we didn't meet you before we left. If you meet Vasu in the
office, don't tell him we are away because he'll think we left him
so as not to pay him. Tell him you haven't seen me and maybe I'm
sick. Beyond that I will not write. Thank you for your cooperation.
Write to us.

See you soon,
Isaac

Three days later, on April 17th, Isaac is already in Lille, 350 kms south of
Nancy. Did he really make that journey, or was the earlier postcard also sent
from Lille? Writing from Hôtel Bellevue, 5 Rue Jean Roisin, 59800 Lille, France

…Yesterday morning I was in a hurry and forgot to leave the
envelope with the 60F with the concierge. I found the envelope in
my pocket, in **Cambrai**, *a city famous for its candies. You will get*
the money tomorrow elsewhere. I'll be back next Sunday. Hope
there is nothing new…

The following day a picture postcard is sent from **Vittel**, 380 kms south of
Lille, but only 50 kms from Nancy, describing cynically the curative effects
of the water it is famous for.

… Am having an Aperitif with Vital water but without Meze[31] *and*
Raki it tastes like shit… What do you know, they say the water is
like wine… that's what they say…and drink the stuff all the time…
I'll have to drink the stuff for 21 days….

And then, on June 12th, at the same time Leon wrote to their mother in Salonica and begged her to write to him and while corresponding with Jeanne about
his business letters, Isaac is to be found again in northern France, returning to
Cambrai, 60 kms south of Lille. Four days later, he sends another card from
Boulogne-sur-Mer, 110 kms west of Lille, a town on the English Channel. As
four days later, on June 16th, he sent a postcard from **Calais** itself, was he trying to get to England? It is very confusing since the very same day he sent yet
another card, this time from Bethune, which is 60 kms south of **Calais**.

… I have business in the area and I don't know if I'll be back
tomorrow. Wednesday I'll be in Paris. If there is something very
urgent, write or send a telegram or phone. I'll ring you twice a
day, at noon and in the evening. You can leave a message with the
concierge at the hotel… I finally got the car on Sunday around
nine and can you believe it, there were problems with the ignition…

On July 7th, Isaac is back at the Hohneck, near Gérardmer. He also sends a picture postcard from **Munster,** a small town only a few kilometres from the mountain. Three days later he sends a card from Hirson, 300 kms north, reporting he is on his way back to Paris. It is quite a journey to be making in such a short time.

... Last night we left Epinal to return to Paris. We went through Nancy and found your letter which contained no news. Instead of going to Paris, I decided to go to Lille and Cambrai where I have business. I ask you Leon if you can deal with these things with the Galeries Barbès.[32] *It is very important that money will be sent to Mr Jobert, a judge at the Tribunal, with a letter asking him to sign the contract with Galeries Barbès... Martha requests that you send her blotting paper.*

Tell Zion to wait 3–4 days because Martha had paid him a week ago... don't give him any more money. You can ask Marcel or the concierge to ask Arnav and I will pay him back. It will be quicker that way. Try to delay the visit to the IRS. Also try and get the letters from Adam Marcel. I plan to come back tomorrow.

P.S.

Do me a favour and tell the advocate Metro Jean, who lives on the same street as me, that I return on Thursday and I'll call him...

Two months pass and Isaac is on the road again. On September 7th, he sends a postcard from Nice, way down in the South of France. He travels to near-by **Grimaldi**, 30 kms from Nice, just west of the Italian border. Both postcards convey little actual information. Two weeks later, September 21st, he is at Malo-les-bains Dunkirk, right on the other side of France, 1,200 kms away!

It is hard to escape the impression that he is on the run, trying to earn money to repay debts and using Leon as an ally back in Paris to back him up. The map of the places he and Martha sent cards from is spectacular. Ninety years have elapsed so any thought of retracing his steps is almost ludicrous but still suggestive... does memory linger in such a way? Would such an investigative journey be what Freud would no doubt think of as a *compulsive repetition complex?* Or perhaps some poetic truth can be found...

The year draws to an end with the long awaited answer from Rachelle Cohen. She is addressing in Solitreo both brothers as she writes in October 22nd but directs her reproach to Isaac for not writing at all.

My dear children,

Since I am not in the best of health, I cannot write at length. I write you these few words so you are not alone. I hope this will not stop you from writing yourselves. I hope everything is fine. How do you see life in Paris? Is it better than Salonica?

You, my beloved Isakino, have forgotten your dear mother who loves you so much and is eager to see you and hug you. If the Lord grants me the possibility to see you I would be very happy.

I embrace you with all my heart. Your mother who loves you to the end of the world.

Best regards to Martha.

A month later, Eli, their younger brother, wrote on November 22nd, not having heard from Leon all that time

... We haven't received any news from you in three months. We all worry about your silence. Mother is very worried and thinks you are sick. I expect we will receive a long letter soon telling us that you are okay. Mother is very worried about the autumn cold and rain and asks you to take care. Here, thank goodness everything is fine, except for mother who sometimes has stomach pains. But Rita takes care of her all the time. Rita, as you know, is in the seventh month, and already prepared all that is needed for the baby. Everyone is waiting for the birth.

I have been unemployed for five months. The company I worked for was closed down three years ago and since then I have been looking for a job without success. Even with the connections we have, I can't find a job. I thought it was good for you to know and maybe consult Isaac.

Dino was conscripted two months ago so he can't help out in the upkeep of the household. Benjamin has to take care of the whole family and since he has the headache of the Meza Franka[33] for Rita's wedding, is really struggling. Mother asks you to visit her uncle because she heard he had an epileptic attack. Uncle David is very ill and probably has a sign of dementia. Mom wants to know what business you're doing now. Write to her... Sam sends you and Isaac his warmest regards...

A letter full of information, concerns and a lot of warm sentiment, as anticipated in a closely knit family which does not allow distance to weaken to family ties.

The mention of Uncle David is a mystery. Nobody alive at present can tell who he might have been. How closely related was he to Rachelle? Was he her brother? And if so, where was he that Leon in Paris was asked to go and pay him a visit?

Had the letters been discovered while Rita and Shmuel were alive, the answers would have been forthcoming. As it stands, there is room for some detective work and conjecture, the tools of the postmemorial researcher...

A possible answer is detected upon an examination of another letter which Leon received that year. In March 1931, Leon received quite an intimate letter from Sarah Benardout, 77 Westwick Gardens, Hammersmith, London W14, which reads as follows:

Dear cousin Leon,

Thank you so much for your letter and congratulations.

I hope you are well.

We were glad to hear that your sister Rita is getting married and is going to Palestine.

We're going to write to your mother in Salonica.

Dear Leon, please write us a long letter and tell us about yourself.

I wonder if you would try to find a young man in Paris for me, as I am still single.

Greetings from mom and dad.

Yours,
Sarah Benardout

Enclosed in the same envelope was a photograph. In the photograph, an older woman and a child are seen (Figure 21).

On the back, a short message is scribbled indicating that it is a photo of Mazeltov and her son. It is signed – David. Could it be the same David that Eli referred to in his letter, asking Leon to visit him? Was Leon expected to travel to London, or perhaps David was also living in Paris? At first, it seemed a far-fetched connection, not least because of the age difference. Nevertheless, it started me searching.

Who were the Benardouts and what is exactly was their connection with the Cohens? Again, nobody alive is able to remember if there was a family connection. Rita's children, themselves now in their eighties, remember only vaguely that there was some connection that Rita had mentioned, but its exact nature remains a mystery.

It took me several cul-de-sac online searches which seem to lead nowhere but eventually a link was found to a rather obscure website set up and managed by Aharon Ben-Yoseff, a former British citizen now living in Beer Sheba, Israel. A message posted on the website was promptly responded to by Ben-Yosseff, a retired lawyer in his early eighties. A meeting was arranged and a few days later, I found myself sitting in front of the man who

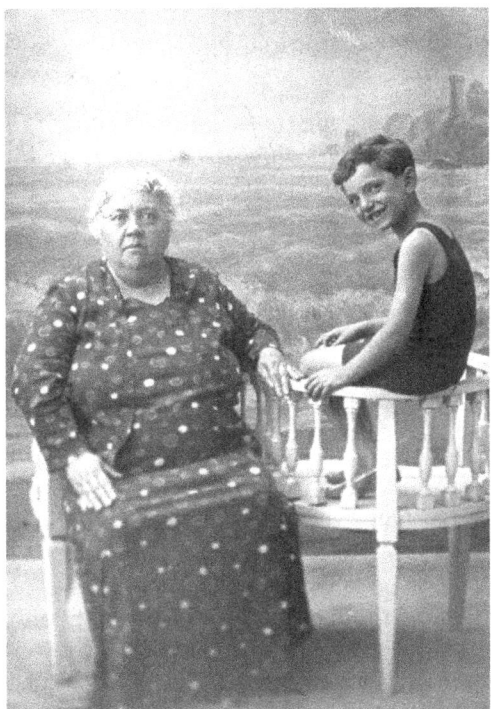

Figure 21 Mazeltov and David Benardout.

may well have been a living relative of the Cohens, though perhaps a remote one, but still, a living person. We met in a café near the border with Gaza, had a few coffees and tried very hard to find out how and if we were related. Though we did not come to any hard evidence conclusion, it was clear that a bond was formed.

Aharon kept mentioning another cousin living in Israel, Marlene Sternbach Benardout from Petah Tikva. From there, it was only a short distance to the discovery that the author of that 1931 letter, Sarah Benardout, was indeed her aunt.

The second letter from the Benardouts which was found in the boxes clinched it. In May 1934, Solomon Benardout, Sarah's brother and Marlene's father, wrote a letter to Leon. Its contents show that the families were indeed in close relations and were blood-related. The letter is occasioned by perhaps the happiest event in the Jewish family register, a wedding. He responds to the news of Leon's forthcoming wedding in May 1934, enquires regarding Rita's wedding which in fact happened three years earlier in 1931 and informed Leon of a wedding of a cousin.

Dear Cousin Leon,

I received your wedding invitation, but I can't write well in French, so I'll write in English.

Dad and Mom were really pleased with the wedding invitation. It was the first time we heard from you after many years.

Mom wants to know when your mother will be in Paris and maybe she will want to come to London for a vacation.

Please write to us and tell us if your sister Rita is now married.

Your cousin is about to get married in August and so is my sister Sarah.

Yours affectionately
Your cousin
Solly

It was soon clear that I have discovered a blood relation, the closest I got so far to finding a real living relative whose mere existence felt like a connection to the memory of Leon Cohen. What had been established was a real link to a past that was thought to have been totally obscured. It was like finding a ladder that led the quest to another level. It was finding a kindred spirit who had been searching herself. It was like two ghosts bumping into one another in the dark and finding comfort in the arbitrariness of the encounter, as if it was signifying a revival, a resurrection. The joy of meeting Marlene and especially witnessing her deep emotions when she recognized the handwriting of that 1934 letter as belonging to her father, was only akin to my own sensations when sitting with Pierre Quillardet in his Rue le Goff apartment, in the same building where Leon, Bondy and their children lived as I will detail in the Epilogue.

From what I have been able to string together, with Marlene's and Aharon's help, it seems plausible that Leon's father, Shabtai, and Solomon's and Sarah's mother, Mazeltov, were siblings. Mazeltov Cohen was born in Salonica about 1878 and married Aaron Benardout, born about 1873. The two married in Salonica and moved to London around 1910, where they had four children: Lena, Solomon, Sarah and Samuel. The Benardout family mostly lives on in London to this date, having left Salonica in time. Solomon's daughter, Marlene, and Sarah's son, Nati Rozenberg were both born in London but are now living in Israel and are therefore my cousins, three times removed.

It is therefore quite logical that in her letters to her sons in Paris, Rachelle Cohen would urge them to maintain contact with the family on their father's side. The two branches of the Cohen tribe in Salonica were able to keep in contact in the years before World War II. When the war was over, that link was severed. These two letters indicate that the London Cohen branch knew of Rita's existence in Palestine. It is not known, and will never be known, whether they had tried to make contact with the only surviving member of the Salonica Cohens. It is a sombre thought, thinking that perhaps no effort was made on either side to renew contact. Marlene Sternbach Benardout, Nati Rozenberg and I have discussed this at length. As neither had ever heard of the existence of the Salonica branch from their parents (Sarah died in 1939, so it is not surprising her son knew nothing, but Solomon died in 1986, which is uncanny as it is the same year of Rita's death), who clearly knew about them, it will forever remain a mystery as to whether any contact was attempted. It is probably safe to assume that both branches of the family were busy surviving, establishing homes and raising their families during the years after World War II and therefore had little time and resources to reach out to more remote branches of the family. And perhaps they tried but frequent moves prevented those attempts from coming to fruition. We know that the Benardouts, for instance, left the Warwick Gardens house soon after Sarah's death in 1939. And the Parentis in Palestine had changed addresses at least a couple of times after their arrival, so it is easy to understand how letters would get lost and the contacts slowly dissolved.

Despite those somewhat troubling questions, it is as uncannily reassuring to know that someone other than Rita's descendants have survived from the Cohen tribe, someone who is still alive and within reach, a blood relative with whom the stitching of this postmemorial tale is still occurring.

1932 – Benjamin's wedding and the economic crisis

What books did Leon Cohen have in his library once he settled into a more comfortable life? Was he aware of the rich cultural scene around him? Was he aware, for instance, that Ze'ev Jabotinsky (1880–1940), the Russian-born Jewish leader and founder of the Revisionist Zionist movement which would eventually become Israel's ruling party from the late 1970s, was living in Paris during almost the whole period that he did? In 1930, for instance, Jabotinsky published his novel *Samson*, which outlined his vision of the reawakening of the Jewish national movement. Was Leon aware of that? None of the letters indicate that, which is strange as his brother Benjamin and even his brother-in-law Shmuel Parenti were Zionist activists and no doubt knew of Jabotinsky's reputation which was becoming somewhat of a personality cult. As well as his political activities, Jabotinsky led a bohemian life and frequented the many cafés in his Montparnasse neighbourhood, like many in the thriving Russian émigré community. Did he come across Henry Miller? He was one of the few Jewish leaders who sensed the imminent danger and urged all Jews to emigrate to Palestine, even by force and in open defiance of the British Mandate. That was also one of the major differences between his movement and the Socialist Zionist movement, headed by David Ben Gurion (1886–1973) amongst others, which took the view that immigration needed to be monitored so as to not upset the British. Jabotinsky was lucky enough, one might say, to have collapsed and died, only sixty years old, on a visit to the USA in August 1940 and did not witness or suffer the fate of the millions of European Jews he sought to rescue.

For Leon, 1932 opens with another wedding of the Cohens – this time of Leon's younger brother, Benjamin, four years younger than Leon, the sixth in the Cohen lineage. He jumps the line and precedes Leon, against the Sephardic custom that siblings are only to marry if their elders are already married. This was soon to be mitigated by the fact that Leon himself was to be engaged. The wedding invitation, printed on a special card was addressed both to Leon and Isaac, still at the rue Richer address (Figure 22). It was to be held on March 9th at the **Synagogue** des Monastiriotes, 35 Siggrou, Salonica at 5 p.m. exactly. The new synagogue was completed only a few years before, in 1927, and its building was funded by the Jewish community of Munastir, Yugoslavia, who had fled there during the Balkan Wars and World War I. It stands today, having survived both the Nazi occupation of the city and the earthquake of 1978. It is no longer the active synagogue of former years and the remaining Jewish community of the present day congregates at the newer synagogue at Tsimiki Street. The bride is Alegré, the daughter of Michel Rousso, at 3 Lyssipou.[34]

Three letters from Leon's brothers, Benjamin and Sami portray quite a complex situation in Salonica. Alongside the joy of Rita's wedding, and Benjamin's and Leon's own engagements, the economic situation is dire. They are forced to beg Leon and Isaac to send money home. That, together with Isaac's continued silence, paints quite a grim picture. The first letter is dated February 10th.

... Uncle Menachem[35] passed away... I feel guilty that it's been a long time since I sent you news from home. You can understand that my time is divided between home, office and my fiancée. If I have some time, I prepare accounts. Now here's news from all of us.

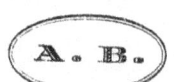

A . B.

M^r & Mme Michel Rousso
& Mme Vve Rachel de Sabetay Cohen
ont l'honneur de vous faire part du mariage de leurs enfants

Alegré & Benjamin

et vous prient de vouloir bien assister à la cérémonie de la bénédiction nuptiale qui leur sera donnée le Mercredi 9 Mars à la Synagogue des Monastiriotes à 5 heures précises.

Salonique, Février 1932.

ADRESSE TÉLÉGRAPHIQUE :
ROUSSO ⬛⬛⬛⬛
3 LYSSIPOU ⬛

Figure 22 Benjamin and Alegré's Wedding Invitation.

First of all, I want to say that Isaac's behaviour can't be excused. If we wronged him in some way, we ask for forgiveness. But I think he must write at least two words to Mom. She certainly didn't do any harm. She is very sad that she receives a letter from you without a word from Isaac. You write that Isaac is not to blame and that made Mama even more sad.

Business here is not good. Local currency is deteriorating with all the political changes.[36] *Eli is unemployed, Dino and Sami are in the army and there are seven people here to be fed, nine including the maids.*[37] *Henri comes in all the time. He sells coffee door to door and earns seventy drachmas a week* (20 francs). *Mother is very tired after Rita's birth.*[38] *You know Rita has given birth to a very beautiful baby girl named Ninette* (Esther's original Ladino name) *three weeks ago. She's fine now...*

I'm waiting to hear from you,

Your brother, Benjamin

The second letter is dated April 9th and is written by Sami. It is written on an official letter headed Nachmias & Mordoch, Fabrics, **5 Siggrou,** the same address as the synagogue.

... I think that Mom should be moved to Paris to be with you and Isaac (who never writes). But Henri, Eli and Dino need to stay here. They are in a bad mood because they cannot find work. Mom wrote to Isaac and told him about the bad financial situation and asked him for help, but Isaac did not answer his mother. He does not understand that he causes her a lot of pain. She is very happy to hear that you are engaged. She also asks me to tell you both that if you could each donate 50–100 francs each month in these very difficult times it would help her. The situation in Salonica is very critical. Believe me, what I sell in the store is not enough to pay the rent. Don't know what will change that. I am the only one working at the moment. We simply don't have enough money.

Yours,
Sami

P.S.

Henri thanks you for the 10 francs you sent, and he will use it for shoe repair. Kiss the evil Isaac from me and tell him we expect a letter from him.

These are harsh times. An even harsher letter arrives from Benjamin on August 20th.

... I read the letter you sent to Henri. You know his wife left him on Passover. The reasons are very simple. She could not stand a husband who can't support her. Maybe we shouldn't write about it at all. He tried so many employment opportunities but was unsuccessful in all. He used to sell women's clothing, hats, insurance policies, bicycles. He worked for his brother-in-law as a coffee salesman. He is constantly trying. It is heart-wrenching. Mother is suffering more than we do. He is living back in the house and it is very hard for her. And yet, since she is now recovering from her hernia, it is also a blessing.

Let me tell you about Rita's wedding. She got engaged two years ago in September 1930. The four of us, Eli, Sami, Dino and myself worked hard and saved about 17,000 drachmas for her dowry. We all gave up basic things like taking care of our teeth so we could give her a nice dowry. It was tough. Then Eli lost his job. Also our uncles didn't give us what they promised. You too, who had thought you may be able to help, did not send anything to your sister, not even a gift. All the expenses of Rita's wedding fell on me. I thought I'd go crazy. Rita was very upset about the dowry because she knew there was no money in the family but her future mother-in-law pressed for more and more. Since then, their relationship has always been tense. I was very nervous. I shared my burden with my employers and they arranged for me a bank loan of 20,000 drachmas. I borrowed from a friend another 5,000 drachmas and he also bought everything needed for Rita's dowry. I now owe 40,000 drachmas, and on top of that I owe 8,000 drachmas to Sam, Rita's husband. I also pay Mom's rent and give 300 drachmas a month for household costs. I do what it takes in fulfilling my duty. I think I am doing the right thing. So, you can imagine why mother is suffering. It's hard making ends meet. Eli and Dino are unemployed, and Henri is maybe unemployable. The value of the currency has dropped and if you can send 25 francs every month, it's not that much it won't dry the sea, but... If Isaac did the same, it would be a great help.

Your brother,
Benjamin

There's a big gap here concerning what Leon was doing during 1932. The tone of the letters suggests implicitly and explicitly harsh times. Leon was still struggling to establish himself as an accountant. The idea of moving to Marseille or back to Salonica is no longer on the table. His family needs him or at least his financial support and he is doing all he can. Even though the economic situation in France during these years was slightly better than in Greece and the rest of Europe, by 1932 it was also hit by the recession, though not as badly as other industrial European countries. But the grim mood that was slowly spreading over Europe was affecting France. The hostility towards emigrants in general and Jews in particular increased, reaching a nadir in 1933 where Jews where no longer admitted into the country. The assassination of the French president Paul Doumer (1857–1932) in May 1932 by a deranged Russian émigré is perhaps disregarded by historians as an insignificant event, but can nevertheless be interpreted symbolically as a sign of the beginning of the collapse of the social order of the Republic and its deteriorating relations to the various immigrant groups, which until then were seen as enriching the lively economic, cultural and social life of the French people. From here, it will only be downhill....

1933 – Arriving in Palestine, hardship in Salonica and a surprise in Paris

On January 30th 1933, a weak German government headed by President Paul von Hindenburg (1847–1934) gave in to pressure and appointed Adolf Hitler as Chancellor. A page is turned in the history book. The lives of millions in Europe and around the world will be transformed. The worst is still yet to come.

If there is one letter to be kept from 1933 that encapsulates the ambience of that time, it is the letter that Rachelle Cohen wrote in Solitreo to her son Leon – the sadness and the sorrow of having her beloved son so far away, her failing health, the longing for better days.

To my very kind son,

I haven't written to you in a long time because my eyes are sick and I can't write. I keep thinking you'll be back in Salonica soon. I want to see you. It's time for you to get married and find a good wife and earn some proper money.

I hug you with all my heart,

Your mother always loves you,

P.S.

Dear Isakino, I hug him with all my heart and please ask him to write a letter to me.

During 1933, Rita emigrated to Palestine with her Zionist husband Shmuel and her baby girl. Thus, she joined her older brothers, Isaac and Leon, in leaving their family in Salonica in search for a better world. Unlike Isaac and Leon, she did find a home where she was able to raise a family of five children and be part of the establishment of the State of Israel. She was not a zealot Zionist like her husband, who was a member of the Zionist movement in Salonica, and she followed him with reluctance and dread. She never stopped missing her family whom she would never see again.

What was that parting like? The journey from Greece to Palestine was taken by boat. Rita, already pregnant with her second daughter, Shmuel and Esther, boarded the ship in Salonica. The following day, they were already in Jaffa Port. Their first place of residence was an old Arab house in Jaffa. They only stayed there a few months as the house was near collapse. Thus began the new chapter in Palestine.

Ines, her older sister, took it upon herself to make sure the different members of the family remained in touch. She was the main protagonist of the following years. It was Ines who kept writing to her brothers Isaac and Leon in France and her sister in Rita. She did that as part of her loving duty, being in effect the head of the family since her mother's health was deteriorating and her elder brother Henri was in a continuous crisis, having lost both his business and his wife.

She wrote to Tel-Aviv and Salonica, trying to maintain as close a contact as was possible through letters, as these two letters to Rita and Leon during February show:

My very dear Rita,

I read your last letter, which came 15 days after you wrote it, and today is the fifth day of Sukkot (the Feast of Tabernacles). *Mom wants you to write as quickly as possible because you are in the ninth month. You know that she is suffering from her eyes and cannot write. Tell Nina (Esther) that Mom is missing her greatly and keeps mentioning her and dear Sam. How is he? Why doesn't he write a few lines?*

Dear Leon,

I haven't read anything from you in a long time… Isaac completely forgot about me. But you Leon, you have not forgotten me. I hope you at least see Isaac. Here everything is the same. The children grow up and go to school but school is very expensive. You have to be rich to give them an education. It's a shame we're not rich. I saw Mom yesterday and she still suffers and misses you. When will we get the picture that you promised us? All the time you just promise. Please talk to Isaac and tell him to remember his sister sometimes! I hope to hear from you. Moise sends his love and the kids too …

Leon's younger brothers, Benjamin, Eli and Dino, each wrote and responded to Leon's letters, when they arrive or pester him with questions when he had been silent for too long. A common theme in all the letters is the increasing concern, and even anger, with Isaac, who did not keep in contact at all. The letters portray a complex and even contradictory picture of what is going on in Salonica. Despite Eli's optimism, the economic situation has not really improved. The prospects of emigrating as a way of bettering their situation are never off the table. And above all, the constant worrying about the health of their mother and sister.

Dear Leon,

... How does Isaac feel, how is his business and how is your business? Are you still working as a free-lance accountant? Mother asked to remind you that you promised that if your business in Paris is not good, you will return to Salonica! I think it's time you came back here. Business is back and I think the crisis of last year is over. Living here is cheaper than in Paris because of the drop in the drachma. With 1500 drachma you can support a whole family. Mother wants you to get married in Salonica. We will have a family reunification.

Watch out for a guy named Carasso who will contact you soon in Paris. Ines says to be careful not to do any business with him. Her husband knows him. Don't give him even one cent even if he says he's going to die of starvation.

Yours, Eli

... I add a few words to Eli's letter... After being discharged from the military, I have not yet found a proper job but am trying with a partner to start a small business of selling toothpaste. I hope to be able to expand this partnership into France and maybe you will have a part in that...

Your loving brother,
Dino

... Sami just shared with me your letter.... You are right that we don't write enough, but nor do you!

After Rita and Shmuel went to Palestine, I helped mother to move... She is not well. The same complaints about her stomach, high blood pressure and eyes. Eli works in a warehouse and earns one-third of what he previously earned. Dino started a small business as a salesman and is very optimistic. Sami doesn't earn much. In a couple of months, he is going to the army. We still have no children. My wife is good and sends her love. I am sure that one day we will all meet again. Henri hardly works and manages to get by selling coffee to relatives and friends. Very shabby. Moise gets along and feels good. Ines does not feel well and must undergo

gynaecological surgery. Not dangerous but it costs a lot of money.
I have a friend in Palestine who might be useful for you as an
agent. I will send you his address...

The situation here is not rosy and I think it would be better if Mom
went to Paris with Dino after Sam goes to the army. Eli will do
fine here on his own. Think about it. I didn't talk to Mom about it.

Your loving brother,
Benjamin

Isaac, the subject of so much concern, spent the year travelling around
France, seemingly totally oblivious and indifferent to the concerns and anger of his family. He sends postcards and telegrams to Leon from Dunkirk
and keeps reassuring Leon that Martha and he will be returning to Paris
soon (Figure 23). Apparently less frantic and less on the run than before, but
still asking Leon's assistance, on the sly...

... If it's very hot in Paris, it is the opposite here. If you want to
give us news, send them to the concierge... Can you do me a favour

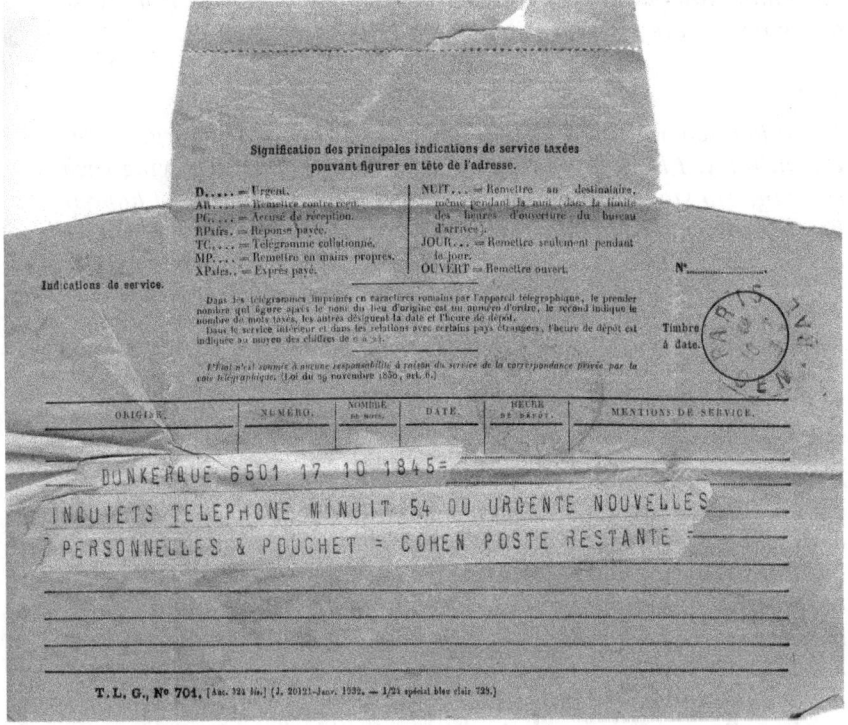

Figure 23 A Telegram from Isaac.

and walk over to my flat to see if there's anything for me?... Hope
to get a letter from you with good news from home and work.
Thank you very much for your help... I think a lot about you and
hope you feel better. I'll be back on Sunday. There is nothing new
here... You must be asking what's going on with us. Soon we will
return to Paris... Sorry for all the trouble I'm causing you...

The year draws to its end. A flurry of letters that Leon kept indicate the big piece of news of the year – his engagement to Bondy Saül. One letter after the other is filled with cries of joy that can be heard from across the continent and over the sea. Letters from Ines are followed by letters from each of the brothers, addressing both Leon and Bondy...

... Mother is very pleased and wants to get a picture of the bride...
She doesn't feel so good. She has stomach problems and high
blood pressure.... You have made a good choice. We received
recommendations about the Saül family. When is the wedding
date?... Why doesn't Isaac care? We have plans to take Mother to
Paris to see a good doctor. Rest and the change of weather may
help her...

.... I know you will be happy with her and she is with you. You have
to love her very much. We only hear good things about her and her
family from people in Salonica... And you, my dear sister, I will be
very happy to know you... I'm waiting for a picture of the two of
you. Too bad we're not together in these times...

How, where and when did Leon and Bondy meet? As they were both of Salonican origin and knowing of the ties that were kept within Salonican Jews in France, it is easy to imagine that they had met or were arranged to meet, *shiduch,* on some social or festive occasion.[39] A possible narrative can be constructed based upon the fact that Leon kept in his box letters addressed to Bondy's father, Vidal, sent to him from a Salonica baker by the name of Haim Tevat during 1930, the year the Saüls emigrated to Paris. As Leon was already an accountant, it is quite feasible that he handled Vidal Saül's business and thus got acquainted with the family. It does not require much imagination to see how the business acquaintance between Vidal and the young, Leon quickly developed to a social contact, where Leon would be invited to the Saüls' household. Many of the photos found in the third box clearly belonged to Bondy and show her in her youth, with her family and friends.

Who were the Saüls, whose re-appearance on my family's horizon led to the discovery of the boxes and made this postmemorial tale possible?

Vidal Saül married Mazeltov Gershon sometime in the 1890s in Salonica. They had seven children, and in more than one way, their story is parallel to the story of the Cohens. It is not within the scope of this book to do justice to their story. They all lived in Paris during the war. Vidal and Mazeltov and three of their children including Bondy, Suzanne and Michel (Menahem) were sent to Drancy and from there to Auschwitz, along with Leon, Bondy and their children. Rosa married Paul Florent and gave birth to Jean-Pierre, Mireille, Jacques and Robert. Rosa and her family survived the war, and it is in her possession that the letters were kept. Mireille's daughter, Marianne, is the author of the memoir quoted below. Two other siblings, Edmond (Solomon) and Clara, survived the war. The Saüls' eldest, Isaac, died at an early age soon after the family emigrated to Paris in the 1930s.

It is perhaps best that the testament of the Saül family is narrated through the words of Marianne Leloir, the daughter of Mireille, Bondy's niece, as written in 2009. She was born and bred in France in the 1960s. This is her postmemorial contribution and her attempt to reconcile with the ghosts of her family.

As a young child, I disliked my mother's mother, Rosa (Bondy's sister who survived the war). *She would nag and shrilly reproach me with reading too much and not doing enough housework. One summer day, I confessed to my father. Concerned as ever with fairness and kindness, he told me about the difficult life she'd had, that her parents, brothers, sisters, nephews and nieces had been killed at Auschwitz; and also how her husband (my beloved grandfather) had died barely a few months after retiring; and how all this had made her lonely and sad; so I had to make allowances… I understood my duty (!) was to love her in spite of her rough surface, to love her because of it, for the sake of the hardships that had made her sour.*

She would cry whenever she mentioned her parents. And I would always feel moved and embarrassed, burdened with this sorrow that nothing ever lightened, that the passing of years seemed never to ease or change in any way. I wanted to console her, but felt such a thing was not possible. As I remember, there was very little explanation; only rage, both absolute and absolutely powerless; the same void, the same yearning, the same senseless absence endlessly reappearing in endless repetition.

When she talked of my grandfather she would also cry sometimes; but then her sadness was blended with fond memories. Whenever I did anything that pleased her, she said: "your Nono would have been proud" or else "your Nono would have told me 'so Hitler did not kill it all off, you see'", or, sometimes, "we are intelligent, that's why Hitler wanted to kill us."

Her relatives had been exterminated because they were Jewish. My grandfather had been proud, and loving, because his wife was Jewish. Being Jewish therefore must mean being intelligent, admirable, loved, and unsafe. I knew very little apart from that. The mystery was attractive – who were they, these people who were loved and admired as well as hated to death? The difference was attractive – they were special. The minority aspect was attractive – on principle, one should take the victims' side.

So, by and by, I came to claim my grandmother's Jewishness for myself – partly out of defiance, partly to make up for the losses, partly in order to feel special. I remember challenging a classmate who had said something about "Jews" (what, I don't remember)... In history class, I mentioned the candelabra with nine candles prominent in the living-room – I had no idea what it was for, apart from affirming one's lineage. In short, I was attempting to become Jewish, because I was not sure I was.

I somehow knew how Jews are Jews because their mothers are Jewish. My grandmother was, therefore my mother was, and so was I.

I believe I knew nothing else. So mine was a dizzying experience of otherness – I was different from others, who were not Jewish; being Jewish was just this – being different; but as that was all I knew, I did not know what it meant, nor what I was. Nor did I even feel sure I really was Jewish, as it seemed to me two generations of non-Jewish fathers could not be lightly disregarded; and also because I could not help being aware that all this – my feeling of being Jewish – was based on emptiness and negation and absence, and, although I was unable at the time to articulate the exact feeling, this identification to nothingness felt vaguely problematic.

I understood it was essential to claim the Shoah – a name that had not yet come into usage at the time. So I got to work learning about it, by asking questions and – mostly – from books. Of course I was appalled by the facts I was getting to know. I would have dreams of us all being taken away from home, in the middle of the night, to be killed. It all both terrified and excited me, and I felt uneasy, even slightly ashamed at entertaining such a murky confusion of emotions.

I was instinctively convinced it was necessary to talk of it all, to remind everyone I came across of the Jews, and above all of their extermination. I was repeating, in my own way, my grandmother's stunned rage, her blind obstinacy in coming back to it again and again; and trying to make sense of it, if only by sharing words about it. Remembering the absent Jews who had been killed in Auschwitz was the only way to keep them from completely vanishing, the only way to fight against the Nazis' will to erase them.

But there was no room in my life for me to give any shape to these attempts; I felt actually unable to restrain myself from talking about it all at the slightest opportunity, but this remained very, very far from what I felt should have been done.

Another difficulty was the adults' reluctance; I particularly remember one discussion, which seemed crazy to me (I was fifteen or so at the time), when my mother and one of my uncles kept saying we should just forget, and I, almost speechless with disbelief, kept repeating "so Hitler won then." I was thoroughly unable to accept that my merely saying this was not enough to make them change their minds on the spot.

When I was twenty I took my grandmother to her birthplace, Salonica – the fantastic city she evoked as the backdrop to the stories from her youth, the city that had disappeared even from the maps and tourist leaflets, in which it has turned into Thessaloniki – ironically, the people who know Greece well seem to consider me a vaguely backward know-nothing with a colonialist streak when I speak the old name; still I cannot bring myself to use the new... The city has spread into a huge modern metropolis, complete with suburbs and industrial plants, traffic-choked and sky-scrapered (or so it seemed to my surprised eyes). As for the Jews, who used to consti- tute by far the largest ethnic/religious community, there were only about twenty of them in the synagogue on Rosh Hashanah, one of the major holi- days... However, we managed to find some recognizable places – the White Tower, "Museum of Archaeology Street" (with the same name, in Greek, and the museum at one end, but a fairly tall modern building loomed where the old family house used to stand), and, above all, we found the sea, the never changing and, yes, "ever renewed" sea...

The trip was followed by unexpected consequences: after my grand- mother and I had been to Greece together, the whole family – my mother and her husband, my brothers and sister, some of my uncles, aunts, cous- ins...– also went. The place, which had been out of reach for over fifty years, had become real overnight; and the land of all our old family tales had become a pleasant holiday resort...

I was becoming an adult. I was getting to know some Jews – which had hardly ever happened before, apart from my few remaining Jewish rela- tives. They generally seemed pleased with my claim that I was Jewish too, though I felt I was exaggerating, if not quite lying, whenever I made it. The mystery lay within my own person, the mystery of otherness: I was Jewish, and was neither able nor willing not to be Jewish, but I did not feel I was fully entitled; above all, I still did not know what it was. Talking with the Jews I met made all these private issues seem more tangible.

Since I was Jewish through my mother who in turn was Jewish through her own mother, would my children also be Jews? The greater and greater distance from the starting point made the notion seem slightly absurd, but then the rule was austerely, soothingly clear, with no room left for half shades. I rapidly put an end to that line of questioning by having children with a Jew whose family was entirely Jewish and, consequently, just as entirely free of that particular kind of soul-racking. My first three children are Jewish through their mother – me – as are all Jewish-born Jews according to the orthodoxy, but they are also Jewish on their fa- ther's side, which (I thought) would preclude the kind of doubts I had for myself.

This also enabled me to experience Jewish things other than painful memories. After my decidedly militant non-religious upbringing, I got through holidays and mitzvoth, took Hebrew courses and biblical seminars, *attended celebrations in synagogues and private homes, submitted to the mikveh ritual of purification, got married under a canopy and had my sons circumcised on the eighth day of their lives. Beyond the religious, beyond the picturesque, I discovered how many-sided Jewishness is, how inconsistent even, in short how alive. I realized that, since I was Jewish, I could be Jewish simply (!) by being myself.*

Essential things changed for me through all these inner shifts and readjustments – but some changes also came from outside ...

My mother's initial response, when I asked her what papers she had that might help me bring official proof of my origins, was sheer terror: "I'd feel like I was sending you off to the slaughterhouse," she wrote. However, faced with a very determined daughter (and her own inner pressures, no doubt) she started off on a long process that finally led to her taking into her own hands the responsibility of memory.

This has sometimes made me feel dispossessed – after all, I used to be the only person in the family who seemed to care about all this, the others ranging from indifferent to downright hostile, except for one source of support, my grandmother, who was ambivalent about it all, to say the least – when I got religiously married, she said "It is all my fault..." which I then took to imply she felt guilty about marrying a goy, though in retrospect she might just as well have meant my marrying a Jew.

Now I feel I have been freed. For my mother has little by little shaped and taken responsibility for the remembering that is necessary for any life to go on its true, subtle, flexible course. She has done so thanks to her specific qualities, her ability to organize, make things happen, meet people, but above all because she is in the right position to do so, as her mother's daughter. I never quite knew what to do with that burden, as in truth it was not really mine. I would not even have been able to say so earlier, and only now fully realize the tremendous tension caused by the false position I tried to hold, struggling to carry on the family history unbroken as it were above the heads of the intervening generation. As if one link (my mother) had been missing from the great chain of life, and I had to enlarge – artificially, painfully – the link that represented me so that the whole might not burst apart.

I am aware, I think, of what it took my mother to face all that hidden pain. I also believe that it may have helped her to (re)establish contact with an important part of herself that had all but disappeared in the camps, along with her murdered relatives – together with her first cousin and play-mate Eliane (Leon's and Bondy's daughter), *who was her age exactly.*

One of my difficulties also lay in my non-Jewish ancestry: how to assert myself as a Jew without reneging on the rest of my inheritance? There was my Nono, who loved his wife, her culture and even her oddities, who loved enough to take it all on as a whole – enough, even, to become part of the family himself, goy though he was: my great-grandmother used to say he might have been a Jew from the North seeing the way he looked... There is my father, who loves life well enough to love it in its variety, to love landscapes from all over the world and to prefer the most exotic faces and voices; who taught me to listen beyond a rough exterior to the sorrows and the richness of lives different from my own... I was lucky enough to have in my lineage men who enabled me, well, simply to exist in the first place, but also, and maybe just as importantly, to achieve some internal unity; their open-mindedness was essential in allowing me to affirm difference without my having to reject them.

I often think of the part their example has played in my evolution, when, after long feeling as though it would be impossible for a non-Jewish man to know me truly, I finally discovered the strange ways of love and let my heart grasp that being among Jews does not itself guarantee that we understand, respect and love one another; I was lucky enough to come upon a goy (The Hebrew word for a non-Jewish person) with a heart and a head that he uses in equal measures in coming to terms with the world, Judaism and his own wife. Without him, without the light of his intelligence and the warmth of his love, neither the present text nor my present existence could have come into being – with their integration of a free, joyful kind of Judaism as well as of the lessons of anti-Semitism.

I have been happy to attend some of the commemorative ceremonies my mother has organized; most notably, I was in Paris with my family in 2003 to officially commemorate Benjamin Cohen, my mother's first cousin (Leon's and Bondy's son), who was killed in Auschwitz at the age of seven, along with his father, mother and two-year old sister, plus his grandparents and most of his numerous aunts and uncles. All this is part of what enables me to go on with my own life, in which I can be just the kind of Jew I am, teaching my children to light the Sabbath candles and sing joyful songs as well as for ever mourning the void left by the loss of those I am now able to call "our kin" – "los muestros."

1934 – Leon is getting married and the quest for socks...

I live a double, *unheimliche* life, when writing this postmemory tale. Most of the time, it is the present time, this particular moment being April 10th 2021, after a turbulent year when the world is continuously struggling with Covid-19. But quite often, and in recent years, disturbingly often, I find myself sinking into trepid daydreaming where my thoughts and feelings are lost in what I imagine was, and still is to me, Leon Cohen's life.

Memories that are not mine keep haunting me. I find myself wanting to follow after any shred of evidence that might lead me to a sign of life. Like a dog sniffing the ground, frantically trying to locate the source of the smell. It is hard to overcome the sense of guilt that not enough has been done in the previous decades. Now, it is perhaps really too late. I know that my mother and her brothers have tried their best to locate all possible data. We all visited the addresses in Salonica and Paris, searched the archives and dug into the digital treasures of the internet. Almost nothing was recovered that could serve as an answer, as a closure, beyond the evidence in the four boxes.

Perhaps, what is needed is a posthumous funeral service, burying the letters themselves and with them to bury and put to final rest the pursuit of this postmemory. Can there ever be a resolution? At the present time, the memory is as haunting as ever. The least I can do is to continue writing this account. This might be the nearest I will ever get to a resolution, to a closure, to finding some rest. Writing is a process whereby to erect a monument to their memory, where others can come and read, come and visit, come and pay their last respects.

Can the memory be buried and done with, along with the physical evidence? In 2019, after a prolonged, emotional complex process of consultation among the Parenti siblings and their children (my generation), it was finally decided that the whole collection should be entrusted to the Yad Vashem Institute in Jerusalem, where it would be digitized, archived and in due course become public for the use of future research. After several meetings with the very efficient and sensitive Yad Vashem professional archival staff members, a visit was arranged, and the contents of the boxes, now arranged in folders, were handed over. A few weeks later, a parcel arrived containing three disk-on-keys, containing all the material, professionally scanned. This handing-over process, which was, of course, documented by me on a video, brought to an end the actual possession of the letters by the descendants of Rita Cohen. It had undergone so many phases: first, after the initial discovery of the first and second boxes, it was put by Rita's youngest son, Benjamin, in special folders with tissue paper separating and safeguarding each document like a precious jewel. Then, after the discovery of the third and fourth boxes, I scanned at home all the hundreds of letters, photos and documents from all four boxes, which were kept in my home, causing both a sense of pride but also terrible dread lest something were to damage the original documents. The scans I had made, I organized into digital folders, arranged by topic and year, translated into Hebrew and English and made available on-line to the Parentis, all three generations of them. Once the actual original materials were taken by the experts of Yad Vashem from me, I experienced both a sense of terrible loss as one would feel after an actual burial and also a sense of relief, as I was no longer the sole guardian of this awesome and tragic family treasure.

The year 1934 opens a period of six years where the triangular correspondence between Salonica, Tel-Aviv and Paris was at its peak. The marriage of Leon in Paris and the move of Rita to Palestine and the births of Zmira, the Parentis' second daughter, re-ignited the need to stay in touch to keep the connections alive. Many dramas took place during those years. There's hardly any need for explanations as the letters speak plenty. I step back and let them tell the story.

On January 19th, Esther Parenti's second birthday, Rachelle Cohen writes to the new couple in Paris.

My two dear children Leon and Bondy,

... I was delighted to see your wedding photo, congratulations and success in business... [Figure 24] I hear that you are working with your dear father-in-law... (Videl Saül)... We all miss you very much, especially Ines who received neither a letter nor a picture from you... If you could buy for me some elastic socks, it would be a great relief. My ankles are very swollen, and I can no longer walk with ease. If you could find a way to send them over with someone...[40]

Six months later, on July 23rd...

... You know, dear, I have not stopped sending you letters...you say you don't receive them... Has your leg healed? Please write...Is everyone okay? Dear Sam, how is business?

Are the two little girls well? Do you take good care of them? I really miss Nina, give her many kisses from me and hug her... I

sent you with Merica two small boxes of burnt Sharope (a sweet
liquid also used as a cold remedy) *and one of Tazikos* (almond).
*Did you get them?... Dear Sam, you know that Rita needs elastic
socks because of her veins... it is a feminine family trait... Please
buy her two bandages and she will put it firmly on her legs...*

Second to her mother, Ines is the central axis in trying to keep the different parts of the family in Tel-Aviv and Paris informed. In one letter after
the other, she pours out her worries concerning their well-being, always
expecting the letters to arrive sooner. Not being able to maintain the close
proximity they were used to, the letters are peppered with news of people that are part of their social and familial circles. It is as if she makes
the utmost effort to make sure that Rita in Tel-Aviv and Leon in Paris
are able to still participate in her life. The contents of the letters often
repeat themselves, indicating the sense of the growing gap in the fabric
of their relationships, missing out on what used to be daily contact. The
joy of knowing that they are all forming independent lives is always min-
gled with the sadness that they are not able to share the mundane details,

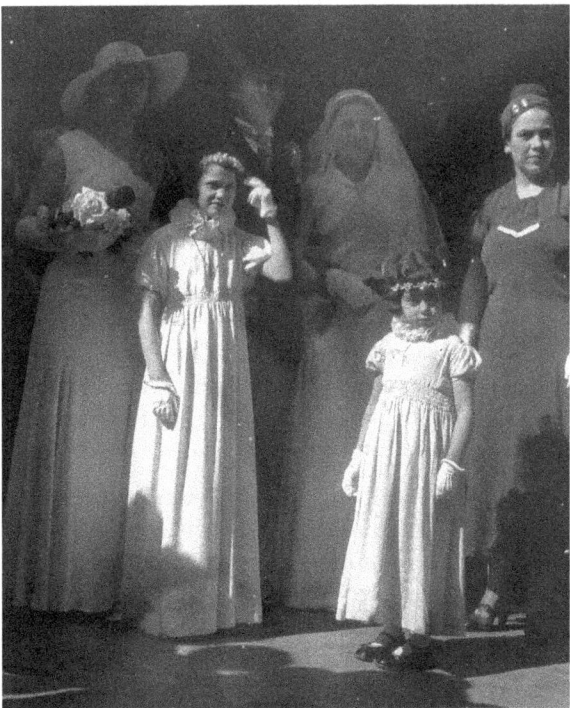

Figure 24 Leon and Bondy's Wedding.

those daily routines that they were all so used to. That ambivalence is most evident when she reports about their mother's deteriorating health, not hiding the fact that the separation from her children is causing her pain.

She writes letters to Leon and Rita on the same day, connecting them thus in her correspondence, almost like having a conference call. In January, she writes...

My very dear Rita,

... I read your letters with pleasure....We wrote a letter of congratulations to Leon for his engagement with Miss Bondy Saül, a good Salonica girl...May God give Leon good luck because he really deserves it... we are very worried about you and Sam... I imagine dear sister that it is not easy raising two babies....

Dear Leon,

I received your beautiful letter and also a few lines from Bondy that made me very happy...my little brother, your letters make me so happy, so proud to be your sister... I need that affection from you, even though it is from a distance... you do not forget me... but, Isaac doesn't care about anyone. Mother is now very sad, locked up at home alone, sick and unable to take care of herself. Forgive me dear Leon for writing these words. It does me no good every time I see our mother, older, alone, missing everyone and especially dear Rita and the little girls (Esther and Zmira)... I would send you a picture of all of us together, but it is very expensive now. We are busy preparing everything for Benjamin's baby. You probably know, Alegré is in the third month... I do everything I can to help Moise, who alone supports us. Especially since Salomon's school is very expensive. This year, he is finishing elementary school. Next year he will go to a state school.

Moise apologizes for not writing to you. Because of his laziness. He is not in Salonica today but wants you to know that he is your best friend and has very good memories of you.

Ines

A few months later, in September, Ines writes a happier letter, having received a photograph of Rita's children and after Benjamin's daughter's birth.

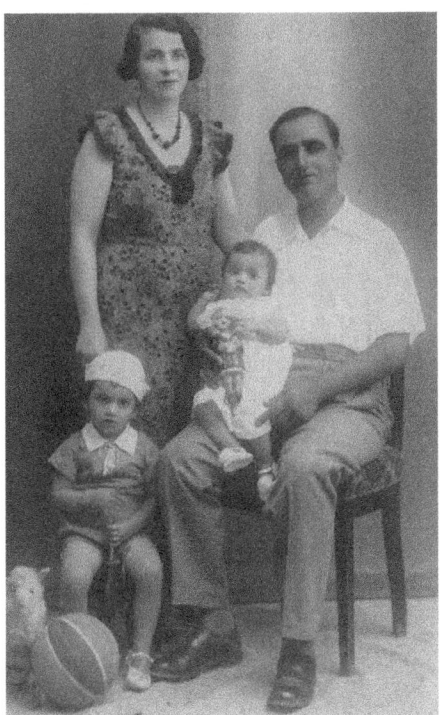

Figure 25 Shmuel and Rita Parenti with Esther (Nina) and Zmira (Martha).

Dear Rita,

With great joy we received your letter with the pictures of Sam and the two girls [Figure 25]... you made us very happy.... everyone looks great, though you look very thin...Nina is very pretty...Rachelle looks lovely, she looks so much like Benjamin's daughter...[41] *But we wish we would hear from Isaac... it was Dad's memorial last week. So sad...I have many things to write to you, dear Rita, but every time I write, I get so upset that it is difficult for me to continue... Moise says that he doesn't even have time to hug his own girls, but sends his love to you...*

Ines

Dear Rita,

I received your letter... you don't say anything about Leon's picture, didn't you get it with the letter? [Figure 26]... Dear Sam,

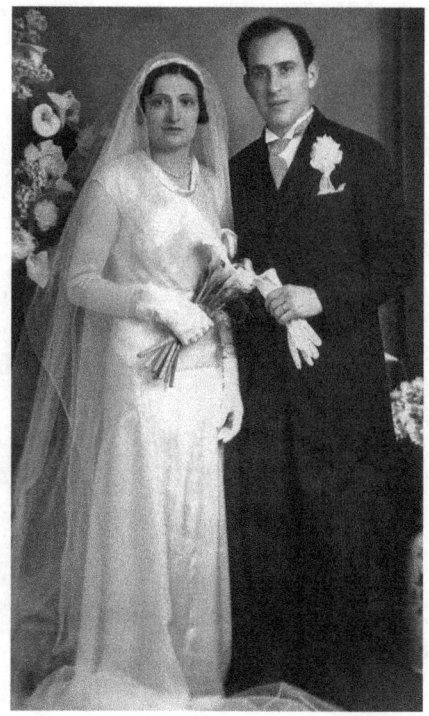

Figure 26 Leon and Bondy Cohen.

*how does he feel? Business is good? May God help him because he
is such a good man...we are all fine, Samiko is looking forward
to his recruitment in two months... How do the girls feel, I have
a great longing for dear Nina...has Rachelle grown properly? In
a few days you will get a picture of Benjamin's daughter. She is
very beautiful... may God give me the right to see your girls. Send
me pictures of you all because I miss you very much. I am always
happy with your beautiful letters... I embrace you with all my
heart...*

Rachelle

*...I write just two lines so you know we're all fine and feeling
good... and Ricetta* (his wife), *my children, Shabtai, Moise, and
Dejo...Congratulations to Sam and the gang* (probably those who
came to Palestine in the meantime).

Henri

*...I was delighted to read that Sam's business was improving...
mother is constantly suffering from high blood pressure...*

Eli

*... You must be angry with me for not responding in time to your
last letter... I am so busy at the store I don't even have time to
go to the bathroom... Alegré and I are not sleeping at night with
Rachelle. Doctor Modiano said when she gave birth the next time
she would have to "sew it", but I am afraid of complications in
these matters.... Some news about my Zionist activities. I am now
President of The Theodor Herzl Society and Sam Shaki*[42] *is the
Secretary...And you Sam, what Zionist work you do in Palestine?*

Benjamin

Another string of letters from Salonica is directed to Leon in Paris. He,
too, is recruited by his brother in trying to help find solutions to alleviate
Rachelle's medical issues.

*... see the prescription that the doctor wrote for mother. We
can't get it in Greece and we thought you might be able to find
it in Paris. It costs 150 drachmas here... If you find it, send it
by registered mail immediately... Take care... you are no longer
writing every month... we want to know the wedding date...thank
you for sending us 500 drachmas... it made mother very happy.
We also received 50 francs from Isaac. Together it's not a small
amount! ... I ordered her a belly belt... the doctor said she should
diet and rest. We have someone living in and helping her so that
she could be more comfortable... Sam is in the army... don't forget
her socks.*

Eli

When the actual wedding date arrives in May, the flow of letters and greetings from the Cohens in Salonica, each writing a letter, is an attempt to
compensate for the inability, again, to participate in the event. As some of
the contents are being repeated, I present here only Ines's letter which spells
out the complexity of Leon's situation in such a happy moment of his life,
experienced far away from his family. Eli's letter, which follows, adds some
different flavours.

Dear Leon,

*I just received your wedding invitation and was very happy... Just
got back from Alegré and Benjamin to help them with the baby
[Figure 27]. Mother can't help much so I go almost every day.*

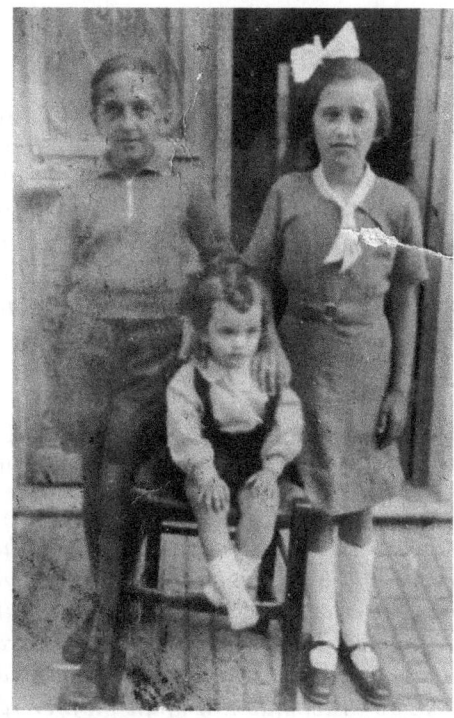

Figure 27 Solomon & Nelly Matarasso & Benjamin's Rachelle.

I fulfil my duty as a big sister... by the time you get this letter, you are already married. Moise and I wish you happiness and prosperity and lots of children. I wish I was there for you too as the older sister because I imagine neither Isaac nor his wife will be the ones to replace us...I would also like to be rich to be able to send you a wedding present, but God does not want that at the moment....

Ines

... The reason I didn't respond immediately is because I injured my arm after an ice-skating incident. I slid and fell on my right side on the iron fence. Today I am already better.... The whole house has been celebrating since we learned you were getting married next Sunday... Dino and I distributed all the invitations you sent. One even went to Rita in Palestine today... Regarding the socks, don't worry I ordered them here...Regarding mother's medicine, you must find another way to send it. It is very important to mother's

*health. I am willing to pay customs expenses here. Forgive us for
the trouble we are causing you these days... As you asked, I will go
to meet Bondy's relatives and write to you in a few days the results
of the meeting and what we will do here on the occasion of your
marriage, with the bride's family.*

Eli

Arranging the reception in Salonica in honour of Leon's wedding coincides
with the celebration of Benjamin's daughter's birth.

My dear brother,

*... We are very grateful to your lovely wife for the successful
change in your life.*

*I wish you both perfect happiness as you deserve. For my part, I
barely make a living. I entered into a toothpaste manufacturing
partnership. I hope this business will start earning soon, but
unfortunately, we lack cash to promote it. I will send you a
separate sample swatch of the ointment.*

*Yours,
Dino*

Dear Leon,

We had a visit from Ms. Zakar today.[43] *We invited her for lunch,
and on that occasion, we also invited Benjamin and his wife Alegré
who live next doors... Naturally, the conversation focused on the
subject of life in Paris, and how the engagement with Bondy took
place. Her visit really pleased us, this is a woman who likes to talk
and speak modestly and honestly... Next Sunday, the reception will
be held at Benjamin's whose home is near...*

*Mother thanks you for the elastic stockings and says you are a
good son... She sends you a jar of your favourite jam that she
made with Nelly (Ines' daughter)... We were very pleased to see
the pictures Ms. Penny brought us from you... [Figure 28]. We
hope that the whole family will be photographed soon, and we will
send you some pictures. You will get a chance to see your growing
nephews...*

Eli

Not only Leon's family are celebrating. A letter from one of Leon's Salonica
friends serves almost as an epitaph to his days of bachelorhood. It is a friend

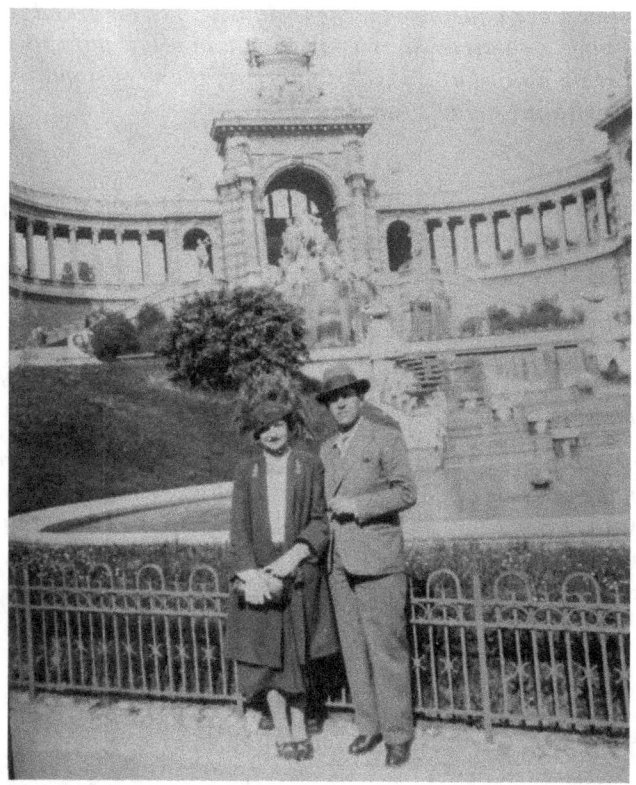

Figure 28 Leon & Bondy Cohen.

who has not written to Leon before, or at least not a letter that Leon kept, and yet, it is a letter written with a collective voice. Even though the writer is unknown, he does mention others of Leon's friends who have written to him in the past, such as Nissim. The letter echoes a time spent as young men, perhaps in the youth movement that Leon belonged to. In the third box was a group of photographs dated 1917, which Leon took with him to Paris, showing him with his friends in what seems to be a field excursion (Figure 29), another group of photographs dated 1919 carry *Bon Voyage* inscriptions from his friends (Figure 30).

Dear friend,

Knowing that you are getting married has given us, as you can imagine, a lot of joy.

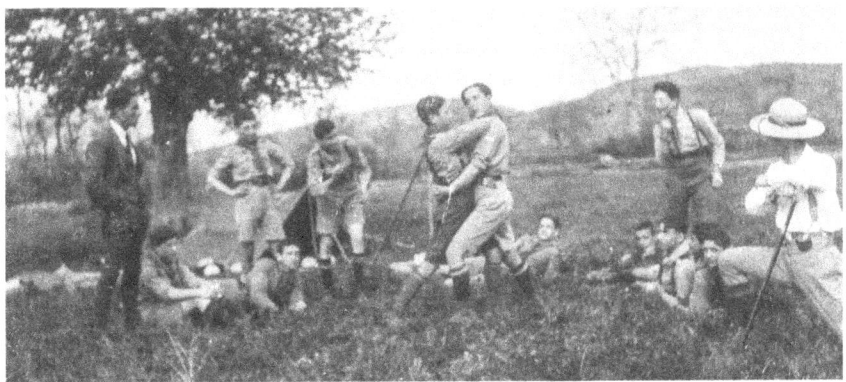

Figure 29 Leon Cohen's Friends circ. 1917.

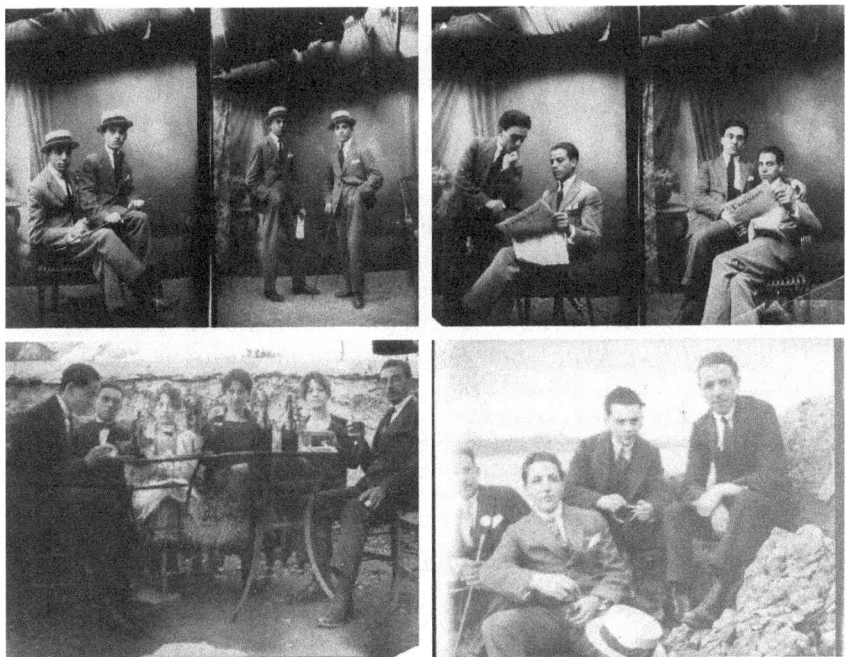

Figure 30 Leon Cohen's Friends circ. 1919.

When we all received your invitation, we were very excited, and naturally remembered the years that we spent with our beloved friend whose picture in our memory remained alive and vibrant despite time and distance.

Here you are, Leon, entering the Family Fathers Club! We wish you and your dear wife, whom we love despite not knowing her, long life, perfect harmony, robust health and good business. The bond of our pact which was broken by Jacques four years ago, is now broken again...Nico and Nissim are clinging tightly to their bachelorhood, but as the years pass, they too will eventually "bury" their bachelor's years, and the Bachelor Square will be replaced by Father's Square.

We often meet with your brothers. They are happy and plan to celebrate your wedding with a small and intimate celebration, which we would love to attend.

Send us a picture but not of your miserable self – have your precious little wife next to you. In return, we will photo the three of us together and in this way we will help you introduce us to your wife...

Last and not least, a single letter from Rita was kept by Leon, imploring Leon to keep her informed...

Dear Leon,

Why didn't you answer my greeting for your wedding? I'm very worried about you. I received your picture and the official invitation and rushed to reply to you with a long and detailed letter. Please my dear brother, answer me and tell me about you and your dear wife Bondy who I did not have the pleasure of knowing.

I send you 2 pictures. One for you and the other for Martha and Isaac. I'm sure you'll answer me soon.

Thank goodness I am always busy, so I suffer less.

Ask Isaac to send me a picture of him.

Rita and Sam

The far-right movement in Europe was gaining strength. Capitalizing on, and fuelled by, the on-going economic crisis and anti-Semitic and anti-government sentiments, anti-parliamentary street riots in Paris were organized by far-right groups, seen by some as a failed putsch, in February, only a few minutes away from Leon's flat on rue le Goff. It was countered by widespread unrest and several riots by left-wing organizations. It all culminated in the deaths of scores of demonstrators on both sides, a solidification of both the right and left-wing parties and the resignation of the president of the Third Republic, the left-wing Édouard Daladier (1884–1970), leading to the formation of a national unity government, including Philippe Pétain (1856–1961) who later became pivotal in the collaborationist Vichy regime during World War II.

As a direct result of the worsening situation in Europe, Jewish immigration to British Mandatory Palestine increased. Due to the restrictions the British government imposed, most of the immigration was illegal. Although Rita and Shmuel were lucky to have obtained certificates,[44] which allowed them to arrive safely in Jaffa port the previous year, most of the arrival to Palestine during the pre-World War II period (1931–1939), amounting to 250,000 people, were illegal immigrants often risking their lives along the journey.

1935 – Births, a death and the origin of the postmemory

As the years progress, I find myself wanting to withdraw and let the letters speak for themselves more and more. As if the postmemory is becoming more and more real and needs less and less my intervention, my contextualizing and my explanations, the letters of 1935 indeed need hardly any explanation or clarification. They tell a complex story of continuing economic hardship, news of pregnancies, births and deaths in the family. A Benjamin Cohen dies in Salonica and a Benjamin Cohen is born in Paris. And in Tel-Aviv, the third-time pregnant Rita is kept away from the news, lest her embryo will be affected by her grief.

The two busy vertices of the triangle were the exchanges between Salonica and Paris and Salonica and Tel-Aviv. Salonica remains the mother city, where most of the family resides, presiding over the extensions in Paris and Tel-Aviv.

The year is cruelly divided between the time before Benjamin's illness and death in Salonica and the time after, which was somewhat alleviated by Leon's Benjamin's birth in Paris (Figure 31).

Ines continues to be the main engine in maintaining the family's connections, not letting her poor health and the fact that she too is pregnant slow her down. Rita and Shmuel are settled in Palestine and now have with them Shmuel's parents and sister, who have left Salonica and arrived in Tel-Aviv. The following letters deserve to be read with hardly any comments as Rachelle, Ines and the brothers deliver in January a testimony of happy and sad tidings, not forgetting the socks....

Dear Rita,

... please answer my letters quickly... mother wanted to write but her eyesight does not allow it. She waits for your letters impatiently... I will continue to write soon as I now have to lie down to rest on account of heart palpitations...

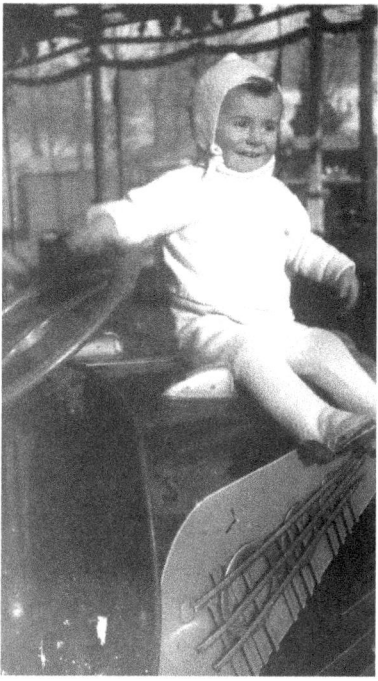

Figure 31 Benjamin Cohen.

Thank goodness I have my mother-in-law who doesn't leave me alone for one second... Did you have a chance to see my sister-in-law and tell her I'm pregnant?[45] *We had a very difficult winter and we survived it with medication and doctors...*

Ines

And in a letter of January 12th, they all wrote together...

... We have received your letter and are very pleased that you are in perfect health. The picture you sent shows how Nina has become a girl and Rachelle who has become beautiful and graceful... You and Sam are thin, that's how it is when raising girls. Don't worry about Mommy, I do my best... She was very happy to hear that you are pregnant... Thank you for the socks but I have to send them back because Customs want us to pay twice of their worth! Maybe you will find a way to get them to us with somebody...

Your loving sister
Ines

... Excuse me Rita I haven't written so far, we're very annoyed by the cold and the constant snows so we can't go outside... Tell me Rita how are the girls? And Bella, you write that she's pregnant? Does she live near you?[46]

Rachelle

... Just a quick word to thank you very much for your concern and the advice about making Aliyah to the Land of Israel... I am ready for that but my wife Ricketa is not a woman who can accept hardship and therefore it is difficult for us to travel...

Henri

... Here the situation for everyone and especially shop owners is getting harder and harder. I hope the girls are fine. They have grown...

Dino

The string of updates is interrupted abruptly by Benjamin's letter which arrives in May.

... I guess you're angry that I didn't write to you...This is because I have been ill for a long time. I couldn't even eat. I felt bad. I had to go to Vienna...

Your brother
Benjamin

A letter that Dino writes to Leon around the same time throws some more light on Benjamin's diagnosis as well as informing us that Bondy had a miscarriage. The letter is written on an official headed letter – Maison Cohen, 14 Venizelos, Salonica.

Dear Leon,

... though Mom is feeling better, Benjamin has been suffering from Myasthenia Gravis.[47] *The main symptoms of the disease are partial paralysis of the tongue which prevents him from speaking clearly, whistling and eating freely. According to Dr Menasche*[48] *here, it is a neurological condition and needs some kind of electric convulsion therapy, which Benjamin receives every day. We hope the treatment will help with God's help.... If you have access to a good neurologist in Paris, explain the symptoms of the disease, and ask him if the electrical treatment is the right thing to do...We are sorry that Bondy had a miscarriage. I hope she is healthy and wish her good health, and soon a baby.*

As for Isaac, I have a bad opinion of him and unfortunately this get confirmed daily. He could write a few words to his good old mother and take an interest in her health.

In my last letter, I wrote that I would send you examples of toothpaste, unfortunately I did not have time to do so. I am sending you two tubes today, one for Bondy. I am now busy in the manufacture of the ointment, but at the moment it not yet successful. In that regard, I visited all the bookstores to find a good informative book but unfortunately, I did not find what I was looking for. I ordered one from Paris through the store nearby your flat, but it hasn't arrived. If you could find me a book on cosmetics that contains all the toothpaste manufacturing data, I would be grateful...

Dino

The letter is followed by a fuller letter from Ines, who tries to put things in a reassuring context.

My dear sister Rita,

... Everything is upside down in Greece these days... you must have read in the press about the recent events, the recruitment of the army, but thankfully everything went back to a quiet state and we won.[49]

And now dear Rita, I want you to read carefully and not be too upset about dear Benjamin who has been seriously ill for four months. It was hard for us to give you this news, but since Benjamin is fine today, I hasten to write to you before you hear from anyone else. The doctors in Salonica did not understand what he was suffering from, and so they offered to send him to Vienna. You can imagine what we went through. We were all like crazy. Dino was the most dedicated and doing all the errands... Finally Benjamin went to Vienna for three weeks and thank God he returned 15 days ago almost recovered but very thin... please send your letters only to me, so that Benjamin does not know that I told you... He is still weak ...

Dear Rita, I made you two dresses from pink fabric for dear Rachelle and Nina so that they remember their aunt Ines who always thinks of her Palestinian nieces and I will send them with the brother of my neighbour Gabriel Dasa who will be there for the Maccabiah.[50] *He promised me to come home to you...*

I hug you.

Ines

Meanwhile, in accordance with the increasing general drive towards emigration to Palestine, Henri decides to try and follow in his sister's footsteps. In a long letter to Rita, he does not mention Benjamin's health and is focused upon his plan to arrive in Palestine.

Dear Sam and Rita,

... Today I have changed my mind and decided that I do not want to stay here anymore. Business is not good and generally life is tiresome. I now think that those who went to Palestine were lucky. Reyna Stromza will be travelling to Palestine tomorrow... I told her to talk to you and Sam, but she did not know if she would go to Jaffa, so she couldn't take the box of sweets that Mom wanted to make for you... I want you to tell me if it is possible to send me an invitation to come to you?

One lawyer told me that if I have someone petitioning for me as a skilled worker, perhaps a locksmith, I will be able to get a permit to travel...Here in Salonica, there is no hope for me, I have to leave...What I earn here is not enough for shoes. I'm definitely ready for any work instead of being doomed here...

I have a plan of leaving here without my family and adopting two boys. I heard that that was a solution. The Zionist agency wants to bring orphans to Israel. The adoption will be fictitious and temporary until they arrive to a kibbutz. The money which I will receive for adoption will allow me to travel. Please look into this matter!

I kiss you with all my heart,
Henri

It seems that nothing came of that plan. As to whether Henri actually tried to realise his plans or whether it just boiled down to him writing the letter, we shall never know. It has been hinted throughout that he was a good-natured man but with little success at actually making his plans come true. And perhaps, the deteriorating state of his brother Benjamin made him stay. Benjamin himself seems to be less worried about his own health than the state of his sister's marriage. In this very last letter he wrote in April, three months before his death, he seems to respond to a letter from Rita where she complained about her marriage. As Shmuel Parenti was Benjamin's best friend and it was he who introduced the couple, he seems to take sides...

Dear Rita,

… I read your letter and was glad to read that the girls are now okay… sometimes you're happy and laughing, sometimes you're sad… I can't understand why you complain. After all you have a good husband… You know, when a girl gets married, her family and her husband become the main thing. He needs to see a happy face when he returns from work.

Don't worry about me, God will take care of me…worry about your own health and your children…

Your loving brother
Benjamin

As far as keeping Leon in the picture, it is mainly Eli's and Dino's letters which provide updates from March to June, usually carrying the very same information that is sent to Rita in Palestine, a mixture of familial and personal with the occasional update concerning local political events, including the failed coup. It is through their letters that we find how dire Henri's domestic situation is, shedding more light on his intention of leaving Salonica and Benjamin's health.

Dear Leon,

I was glad to read your last letter, and I apologize for not answering before, but I think neglect is a family trait, so this is a draw between us as you don't write so much either…

You say that business is not bright, neither is it here. The crisis is still going on, despite our efforts we can barely make a living.

You asked for details and here they are…After 18 months of idleness, I was able through some friends to get a factory job back in September 1932 with a daily salary of 40 drachmas. I put up with this wretched paycheck for the obvious reasons. Later I was transferred to the offices and now I earn 2500 drachmas a month. My work is in correspondence and statistics, it's a good job, I'm satisfied, and I hope to be promoted.

As I told you in my last letter, thanks to our care, Mother's health improved. Your proposal regarding coming to Paris with her and trying to find a bride there for me is good, but unfortunately impossible at the moment… I can't just quit my job in Salonica and seek my luck in the wild… I did think that Mom would make a short trip to France for the change in atmosphere.

I'm glad to tell you that Sam got his job back after he was released from the military. Unfortunately, his salary is very mediocre, barely enough for him alone, but we have hopes for the future. Although Sam is educated and studied mechanics, he cannot find a better job with a higher salary...

Dino will write you a separate letter that I attach to this letter.

Eli

... Benjamin has returned from Vienna and feels very good... he continues to take two pills of Ephetonine once a day.[51] He is able to eat, drink, talk and stroll as before. The professors in Vienna assured him that he was perfectly healthy after the X-rays were negative. Uncle Sam took care of Benjamin when he was in Vienna.[52]... recent events have caused us great fears but now, after the failed coup, it all disappeared like magic... But let's talk about the family...our brother Henry is in distress with his family. We help him as much as we can with our meagre means (Henry eats with us every day) but unfortunately we cannot help him much longer... Ines' Moise barely earns enough to get through the month... Sam will be recruited again very soon...

About the book I asked you about. I found the address of a shop in Lyon which might have it! And it only costs 6 francs. The address is: Perfume Moderne Librairie, 15 Rue Constant, Lyon.[53]

I thank you for the trouble I am causing you, and I hope I will be given the opportunity in the future to repay you.

Kisses to you and Bondy,
Dino

... We were sorry to hear that dear Bondy's pregnancy is putting a strain on her...[Figure 32] According to Mom there is no room for worry... This type of pain is often said to occur after miscarriage... Benjamin is slowly getting better... It's been a year since we received a letter from Isaac. Mother is very sad about his long stubbornness... About the prospects of setting up your business in Salonica, I can tell you without hesitation that I am completely with you. It is true that business is not so good, but with some luck you can get along modestly. We talked to your friends here about this, and they said they would write to you directly and give you their opinion. I know the matter is very sensitive...

Warm kisses,
Eli

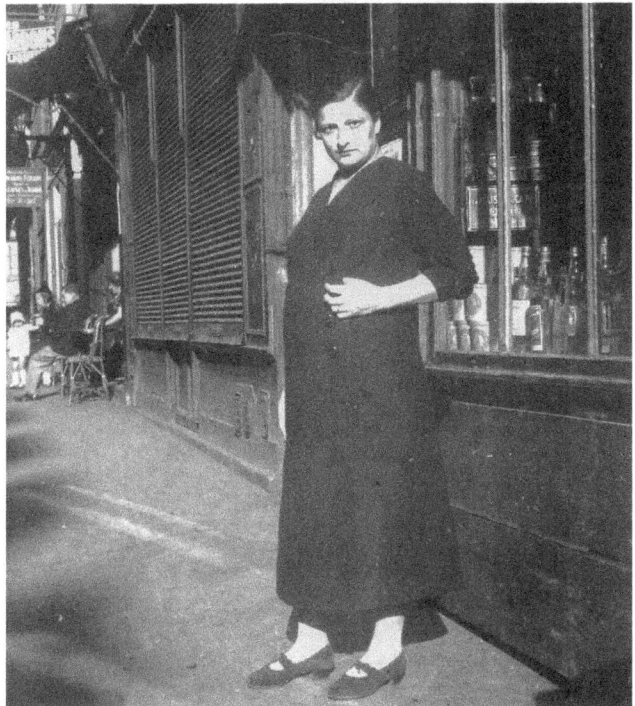

Figure 32 Bondy Cohen.

A few days after that last letter from Eli, on July 7th, Benjamin dies. As he had been the president of the Theodore Herzl Zionist movement in 1930, the local Jewish press in Salonica puts out notices of his death (Figure 33).

The public recognition of his death does little to mitigate the loss to the family, as Ines writes to Leon on July 27th.

Dear Leon,

… A heavy disaster has happened to our poor family, our dear beloved Benjamin is dead…We are lost for words to express our deep pain. Benjamin is gone after an extremely difficult eight months misery without being able to eat, swallow, talk… our poor brother was really tortured…It is very hard for me to write all this.

Throughout the winter, I constantly consulted with Salonica's best physicians, who said after the first diagnosis that his condition was

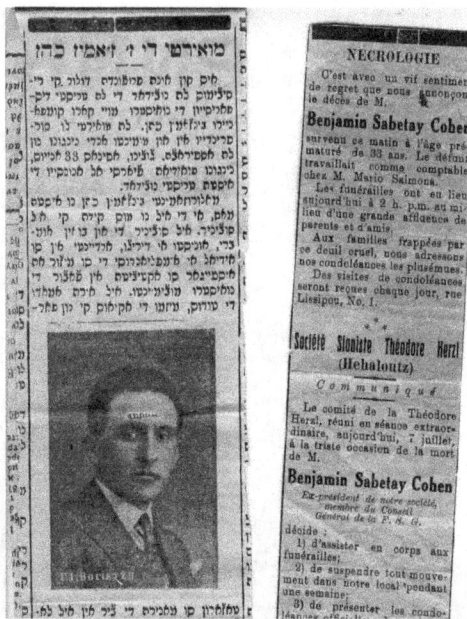

Figure 33 Benjamin's Death Notice.

extremely difficult... I asked Eli to give a donation in his honour to "Matanoth Laevionim (Gifts for the Poor)"[54] during the memorial service of your father-in-law Isaac Saül[55] ... I saw Bondy's aunts... And how is Bondy? I hope that soon you will give us the gift of a good son who will named after our good brother...

Ines

Ines' letter to Leon does not mention Benjamin's wife, Alegré, or their daughter, Rachelle. The mention of the Saül family, on the other hand, shows the strength of the ties between the two families. As Benjamin was a public figure in the local Jewish community, their grief is shared with others. This made even more urgent the need to make special efforts to hide the fact of his death from Rita in Palestine. As she was pregnant with her third child (Shlomo), her family is concerned that if she would know, her grief would harm the pregnancy. The deep emotional tie between Rita and Benjamin was evident in the last letter he wrote to her. So when Ines writes to her in September, two months after the death, she is uncharacteristically brief. The news of Benjamin's death reached her husband, Shmuel, Benjamin's close friend, who was ordered to hide his grief and not tell his wife anything.

My dear Rita,

... I don't know what to think about what you didn't write...You
probably don't feel so well at this stage of your third pregnancy...
Leon wrote to me that Bondy is in the seventh month...

Ines

Leon himself was also asked not to share the bad news with his sister. When
he writes to Rita in November, he focuses upon Bondy's pregnancy. This is
the thirteenth letter in the collection written by Leon himself.

Dear Rita and Sam,

... Bondy is about to give birth in the coming days... we will let you
know as soon as it happens. At the moment, she is feeling well...
It is very sad that we are so scattered, some in Salonica, some in
Palestine and some in Paris. Let's pray that someday we will all be
in one place, happy together. Did you get our wedding photos? We
hope to see a picture of your new baby soon... Please tell us what
is happening to you...Why did you leave Jaffa? Are you happy in
Tel-Aviv? We are told that life is good in Palestine and especially
in Tel-Aviv. But it's very difficult to emigrate to Israel.

Leon and Bondy

A few weeks later, and Bondy gives birth to her son, bearing the name of his
deceased uncle, Benjamin Cohen. The couple receives many letters of congratulations, all tinged with sadness and caution lest Rita finds out about
her brother's death.

Dear Leon,

... I was so happy to hear that your little son was born, I can't find
the words to express my huge joy... How is Bondy? I expect a long
letter from you soon...

Ines

... Dear Bondy, many kisses from me. God bless you and thank you
for giving the boy the name of Benjamin...

Rachelle

A month later, Rita herself gives birth to a son, Shlomo, in Tel-Aviv. She
still does not know of Benjamin's death, but her letter to Leon shows that
she is suspicious. What should have been a very festive event, the birth of a

first-born male child in a Sephardic family, is clouded with the sadness of the distance between the families. The cloak of silence surrounding Benjamin's death is particularly heavy. Why is mourning so feared?

Dear Leon,

... Rita also gave birth to a son (Shlomo) about three weeks ago, but he has not been circumcised yet because he is jaundiced. If you write to her, don't tell her anything about Benjamin because we still hide the bad news from her... As for the conflict we have with Benjamin's father-in-law regarding his inheritance, I will update you in a few words: Benjamin deposited a certain amount in the bank of Athens in a safe deposit box. This money came from his wife's dowry which was partly used to renovate the house. The keys to the safe are currently in the hands of Mr. Bono who claims that according to Jewish law this money goes to Alegré. But Greek law does not allow Alegré to use it yet... We want to ensure at any cost that Rachelle will inherit her share...

Eli

...Mother is especially happy. As soon as we announced the good news to her, she cried out, "It's Benjamin who was reborn through Leonico who loves him the most..."

Dino

In December, Rita writes to Leon, still not knowing of Benjamin's death but clearly suspicious...

Dear Leon and Bondy,

... I was so happy to hear about the birth of the little boy... I'm very sorry we are so far away from each other.... I ask you, my dear Leon, to write me the truth about Benjamin... I am not a baby that you can hide things from, have mercy, my dear Leon and answer me honestly when you receive my letters because I am suffering... I have to tell you, my dear brother, that my baby was sick and he was circumcised only in the second month...I was sick for six weeks, tell me exactly what happens because I am told that Benjamin is still sick with a cruel illness and maybe paralyzed and that he cannot write... I want to know everything that happened to my dear brother...

Rita

This exchange of letters is uncanny in nature as it exposes an underlying familial assumption concerning Rita's ability to mourn and could have been perceived as a warning of future events. It is true that the death of a beloved brother would be a blow to anyone, but the measures the Cohens in Salonica and Paris took to hide Benjamin's death tell another story. I suggest that the family's fear of the impact of the bad news suggests a perception of a deep underlying fissure in Rita's psyche, a fissure which was to magnify to dramatic proportions when she realised the deaths of all her family in the Holocaust, seven years later. For me, the extra measures they took are the very same measures she herself was not able to put up around her terrible grief, thus creating underground shock waves of the deepest sense of loss that affected her children and her grandchildren, penetrating into the depths of our unconscious.

I am not suggesting any mystical explanations but rather relying upon a collective interpretation of the psychoanalytic notion of *repetition compulsion*, whereby an undigested, and perhaps indigestible, psychic phenomenon, as in unprocessed and unacknowledged trauma, creates *a psychic lacuna*, where the repressed emotional affect is so charged up as to project itself in the most uncanny ways. I suggest that the compulsive drive in which I, and many other second and third-generation individuals, have to explore the ways in which the Holocaust has shaped our lives, is to do with such a projection of unprocessed traumatic materials.[56] Hopefully, this book is a creative outcome of that postmemory drive.

1936 – Riots and mourning

August 1936. Hitler writes a memo to Hermann Goering (1893–1946), outlining his grand plan: the greatest danger Germany is facing is world Communism and, in its very heart, the Jews. It is then that his anti-Semitic tendencies become virulent. Once the enemy is clearly identified, the way forward is clear. Having remilitarized the Rhineland in March, Germany is set upon a clear course of domination of Europe.

In Palestine, March sees the beginning of the Arab Revolt, which will continue until 1939. Some would say that it has not stopped since. Its aim is to stop the open-ended Jewish immigration into Mandatory Palestine. The establishment of the Arab High Commission by the Mufti of Jerusalem sets the course for organizing the national aspirations of the Palestinian Arabs.

Fewer letters from Paris survived from this period. The narrative of the years leading to 1942 is mainly based upon the letters found in Rita's box from Salonica. The fewer the letters are in number, the more powerful I find their impact to be. I let them speak for themselves more and more. I summon the ghosts of the Cohens from beyond the grave to tell their story. The details become scarcer and yet, somehow, in an uncanny way, the outlines of the stories become more and more stark. I find myself wanting to withdraw to the wings of the stage and watch the events unfold, undisturbed. Do I harbour some infantile wish that if I interfere less in the narration, perhaps its course would change? Can there be a different outcome than the one I know had taken place? I see myself as a traveller edging towards the end of the journey. With each step, I shed another layer. When the end arrives, there will only be a skeleton there.

In January, six months after Benjamin's death, Ines finally finds the courage to write to her sister and share the grave news.

Rita my dear,

... I promised to write to you at length after the birth of Solomon, but since you were sick and had difficulty handling him, I wanted to wait a bit longer... I have no more courage to hide from you the

disaster and the misfortune of our family.... Dear Benjamin is no longer with us... after eight months of suffering he was admitted to the hospital and after 14 hours he died, on 7.7.35.... Me and Mom were there at 6 am with dead Benjamin...I ran full of tears screaming through the streets...

I hug you all and especially Salmonico (Rita's newborn's nick name).

Don't worry about Mon, she feels better, but mind you, it is not the doctors who will save her, anyway...it is costing us a lot of money, the doctors are stripping our skin... we decided to go to the cemetery and visited Benjamin's and our father's graves... we miss him so much, we lost him forever... Not a day goes by and not a minute without mentioning him... Especially when I see poor Reschelika (Benjamin's daughter)*...I cut her a suit and I embroidered it so that she could wear it for Passover. If Benjamin could see her, he would have been happy...I see from here that your eyes are full of tears, but as you say, tears are comforting.*

Ines

The news of the Arab Revolt reaches Salonica in May.

Dear Sam,

... thank God you succeeded in time to move to Tel-Aviv and that your home in Jaffa was not burned... I imagine what bad times you have been through, but for a moment I did not doubt that you would manage well, knowing you would not lose your coolness. I am glad you intend to settle in Tel-Aviv, so you will be safer and not subject to Arab attacks...the main thing is to be safe... Do you see this problem resolving somehow, because it harms business? Do you ever think of returning to Salonica?

Sami

Ines writes to Rita again on June 29th and shares her news. It must have been a relief to be able to write openly to her sister in those hard times, but also the good news of her son's Bar-Mitzva.

Rita my very dear,

...For the past month, I no longer wear the mourning clothes in memory of Benjamin. It's now been a year... may the rest of the brothers live long and never mourn again... our affection will always remain for beloved Benjamin...Dear Rita, I think of our

*brother Isaac who hasn't written to me since Purim... I wrote him
a long letter and asked if he could lend me some money to take
care of my teeth... But I received no reply from him... I wanted to
be near you to talk to and comfort me, but here we are... Salomon*
(her eldest son) *asks a lot about you these days that he will soon
have his Bar Mitzvah...*

Ines

1936 in France – Léon Blum (1872–1950), the Jewish leader of the French Socialist Party, became the Prime Minister of the Popular Front Government
until 1937. Having been politicized by the Dreyfus Affair at the end of the
nineteenth century, Blum introduced significant economic and political re-
forms during his days in office. After the French surrendered to the Nazis in
1940, he was falsely tried and sent to Buchenwald concentration camp. After
the war, he returned to France and helped to form the Fourth Republic.

Leon is being kept updated as well. As he already knew of Benjamin's
death, he is consulted about legal matters concerning Benjamin's will as
well as the continuing update about his own son Benjamin and the inevitable complaints about Isaac's lack of communication. The letters from January to December need no further explanations. They paint in stark colours
the grim economic situation is Salonica. The unrest in Greece did not ease,
and the elected government was unable to rule. In August, a military regime was established by General Ioannis Metaxas (1871–1941), backed by
King George II (1890–1947). The military dictatorship lasted until Metaxas'
death in 1941.

January

My dear Leon,

*... I was glad to hear that the little one was fine and that the Brit
(circumcision) went well... Tell Isaac I'm surprised I haven't
received any letter from him so far and I really need a letter from
him...*

Rachelle

Dear Leon,

*...I would like to update you about Benjamin's inheritance... we
have to wait five years before it is resolved by law...Mom had the
flu for a few days and she is recovering...*

Eli

March

Dear Leon,

... You are right to complain about our silence...Mother still has high blood pressure... The doctor says this is to do with the grieving... we cannot prevent this after Benjamin's miserable death... she is happy that the baby is feeling well and that dear Bondy is feeling good... we thank you very much for what you have sent...

About fifteen days ago I received a letter from Rita and she very much misses Benjamin. I gave her all the information about our brother's death. Please write to her, she is very lonely and sad... I wrote to Isaac two weeks ago and to this day I have received no reply from him, why does he not answer my letters? Is he really not interested in us? Go visit him, tell him I'm suffering...

Ines

April

Dear Leon,

... We moved again...We are very concerned about Rita and her family because of the riots in Palestine. They say a lot of houses were set on fire by the Arabs and the entire population of Jaffa fled to Tel-Aviv. We hope nothing bad happened to Rita. We wrote to her yesterday and asked her to answer us as soon as possible...

Eli

October

Dear Leon,

It's been three months now since we heard from you... Mom doesn't understand the reason for your silence. Fortunately, Sam's son, Isaac Bourla, came to visit us and gave us news of all of you and also gave us the picture of how cute and precious your Benjamin [Figure 34].[57] *He is a wonderful boy but mostly he does not look like you, he must take after Bondy's family... I went back to work a while ago, because living in Salonica is very expensive, especially the education of my dear children. By the way, I need to ask you for a little favour... for my work, I need new embroidery journals which cannot be obtained in Salonica...Maybe Bondy can help to find them...*

... What is happening with our dear brother Isaac, who for 20 years has not communicated properly with us...it took the death of poor Benjamin for him to remember us briefly and since then nothing... We wrote to him several times, but he never answered. If I were rich and sent him presents he might have thought of his sister Ines. But what can you do.... "out of sight out of mind"... Eli, Dino, and Semico try very hard to make Mother's life easy. But this involves spending money on doctors, on medicine, diet, and so on. Especially after the passing of our poor brother.

We understand that Henri Bourla[58] told you that Mom lives with neighbours. It is no shame to live in Salonica, where the rent is high, with others who are not family. There was no other choice. The house is not so good, not comfortable, but for now there is nothing to do. I also live with neighbours...I would like a private apartment, but then I could not send the children to school... Luckily, Henri Bourla did not come to visit me yesterday because then he would see that I also live with Moise's family ...Moise has

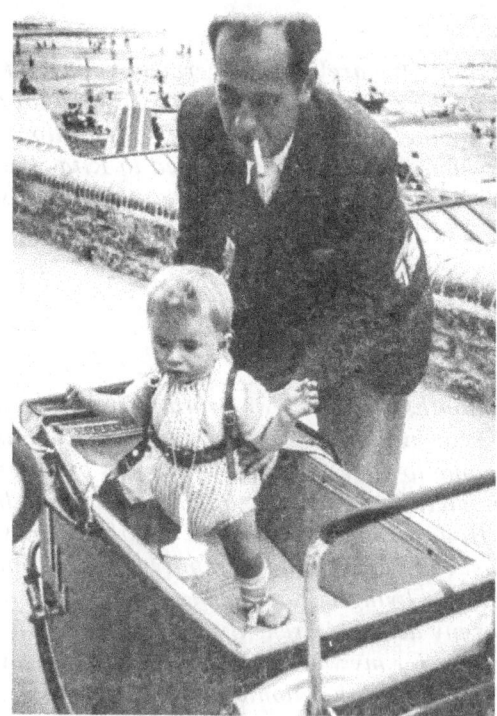

Figure 34 Leon and Benjamin Cohen.

been ill for a while, he is suffering from the stomach, the doctor says he has cramps, and it causes him pain. He also suffers from vomiting. For the past three weeks he has been on an acute diet. You can imagine how it is...

Excuse me for sharing all this pain with you, I know it makes you sad... Thank you so much for the embroidery magazines... they are very good...

Ines

December

Dear Leon,

Finally, after a long, sad wait, I received a letter from you... I hope you're all in good health, is everything okay? Are you hiding something from me? You don't have to hide anything from your big sister, I'm ready to hear everything you have to say, whether the news is good or bad... the sorrow is still deep in Mother's heart... My lovely little Nelly has been suffering from a heart disease for several years, probably because of her poor diet. Last night she had a strong ache and I thought I had lost her. The doctor said she must avoid all activity other than her studies...You imagine what stress I'm under these days... She is beautiful and intelligent, but very sensitive, cries easily... Benjamin appeared in my dream... I often dream about him... I'm also constantly worried about Rita, since she moved to Palestine. Since Nelly is ill, I have no time and desire for another child...

Ines

Rita and Leon themselves exchanged two letters during the spring of 1936.

Dear Leon,

How are you? And how are your dear wife and baby? I don't know how to write this horrible letter in which I have to talk about our dead brother... What a shock for me when I found out. In my stupidity I was crying about his illness while he was already dead. We have lost the best of us. The good heart of Benjamin was lost to us. Poor mother. I don't know what to write and how to ease her suffering... You, too, like me, suffer the brutal loss... It is true that my marriage is successful. Sam works hard and is a good husband (all this I owe to our dear brother) but nothing can fill the hole that opened in my heart. He left a cute girl. The poor orphan stayed with her mother with these bad people, the Russo family. Bad people and big stingers. Ines writes that the little one doesn't feel well, Sam wants to send her something. And your little Benjamin, how is he? How old is he now?

I send two pictures of our family, my three children, my husband's parents, Sam and me [Figure 35]. One picture for you and the other for dear Martha and Isaac.

Goodbye

Rita

Dear Isaac,

You don't write to me anymore, why? After the death of our dear Benjamin, we should have become closer. You hardly knew him. I assure you he was the best of us. Do you cry when you read my letter? I don't know what to write to you. Write me some words and tell me about you and Martha....

Rita and Sam

A couple of months later, on May 22nd, Leon and Bondy respond

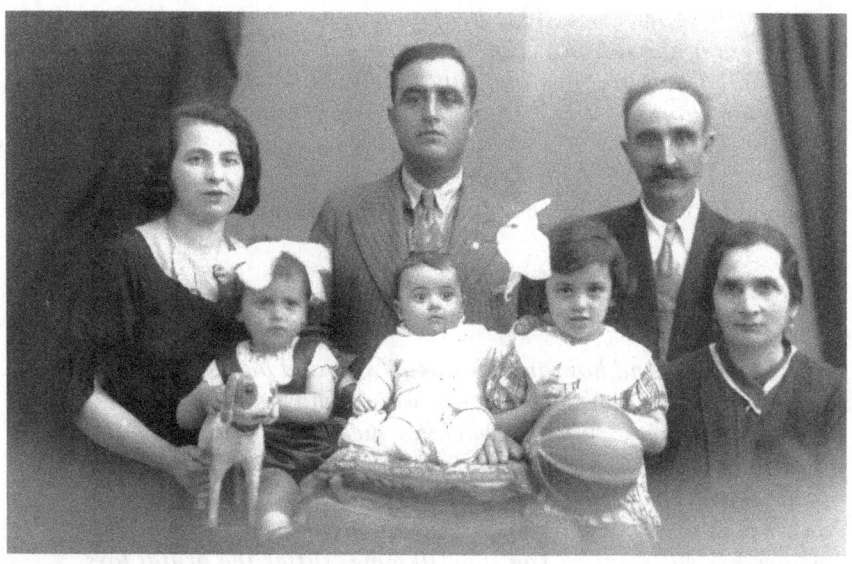

Figure 35 The Parentis in Palestine. Top (Left to Right) Rita, Shmuel and Shmuel's Father. Bottom (Left to Right) Zmira, Shlomo, Esther and Shmuel's Mother.

Dear Rita,

*... I was hoping to get some news about what is happening to you
in Palestine...What is your situation today? How do you feel? Are
you in a war? Do you live away from your mother-in-law? Does
Sam's business suffer because of the situation which seems more
and more dangerous according to what the papers here say?... I got
the pictures, the kids look cute and they seem to get along well. Are
Sam's parents the ones who are in the picture as I think? If so, they
are not completely unfamiliar to me as I seem to recognize one of
my fathers' friends in Salonica. He must be Sam's brother or cousin.
Here, Bondy and I and the baby feel very well, Bondy continues
to breastfeed Benjamin.... We celebrated his first six months on
May 10 with his first tooth. He already has a second tooth...his
mother spends a lot of time on him... Although it is not easy to raise
children here. We will not be able to have more children soon... it's
very cold here. It's not like Tel-Aviv, is it? My Bondy has a very
good friend in Palestine, Sam Shaki who works for Singer. If you
meet them, please introduce yourself to them from us...*

Leon

Dear Rita (and her parents),

*Without having met you, I would also like to thank you for the cute
picture of the whole family. We'll send you ours soon....Here it is
always the same, working hard and trying to earn money as it is
everywhere else...*

Sincerely
Bondy

And Isaac? He seems to continue his search. Is he really oblivious and indifferent to his family's pleas for news? In his October letter, he seems to be on
the verge of a new business venture, again asking his brother to support him.

Leon dear,

*The rain caught me here... is there no more news? I will open the
restaurant on Rue Lafayette probably on November, it's almost
certain... I really want to see you...Regarding merchandise, we
must buy everything wholesale through your in-laws, but it must
all be discreet. We will buy vegetables in Les Halles. We will keep
the accountancy and records separate. Please write something...
everyone is complaining about you. You must tell your father-
in-law not to repeat anything I tell you, he has a big mouth. He*

must not mention the jaundice and thus let my partner regret the whole business. How's Benimino? And Bondy?... Do you have any information from Mama? I want to send her a coat, but I don't have her address...

Yours Isaac

A few years after the boxes of letters were found, another trip was made to visit Paris. The main purpose of the visit was to meet the descendants of the Saül family, and to take part with them in a memorial service held in honour of the victims of the Holocaust in Paris. Small plaques bearing the names of the dead children, including Benjamin's, were placed in the schools where they had studied. It was a very moving experience. The Parentis also went to search for Isaac's restaurant on Rue Lafayette. There was a restaurant there still and the proprietor even co-operated enough to say that he remembered that he had bought the shop from someone who remembered there was a Salonica Jew involved once. It is quite possible that he was "remembering" that out of the kindness of his heart, seeing how much the Parentis were desperate for any kind of information. No official record was ever found about Isaac's restaurant. Furthermore, when the Parentis and the Saüls wrote to the *Commission for the Compensation of Victims of Spoliation Resulting from the Anti-Semitic Legislation in Force during the Occupation (CIVS)* in 2008, there was clear evidence of Leon, Bondy and the Saül family, and a small compensation was indeed given and divided among all the family members (amounting to about 300 Euros each), but no trace whatsoever was found of Isaac, Martha or anything they could have possessed. As mentioned on p. 29, a second attempt has been made recently.

1937 – Sam Cohen – too poor to wed

Fewer and fewer letters are available as the narrative progresses. Perhaps, the Cohens are too busy dealing with the worsening conditions in Salonica, Paris and Tel-Aviv. In Palestine, the British government published a report recommending the end of the Mandate and the division of the land between the Jews and the Arabs. The Arab Revolt continued and reached a critical point with the assassination of the British District Commissioner for Galilee, Lewis Yelland Andrews (1896–1937). In retaliation, the British government banned all Arab nationalist activities. Illegal Jewish immigration into Palestine continued, and many new Kibbutzim were established.

Was Rita really planning a visit home as is demonstrated in Ines' letter to her on January 31st?

Dear Rita,

…We were very pleased to read that you are planning to come to Salonica this summer… I'm pregnant, in the fifth month, and it's quite difficult… Moise will do a gastric radiograph today, apparently he has ulcers, he has already received various medications and injections. The treatments cost 2000 drachmas!

Your sister,
Ines

A couple of months later, on March 9th, Rita receives a collective letter written by Ines and Sami, who will become the protagonist of 1937. No mention whatsoever of the planned visit. This is the first disappointment of the year, but it does bear some good news concerning the situation in Palestine.

Dear Rita,

… What's going on? What is the reason for your silence, is everyone okay? I hope you have received both of my letters, dear

*mother is very worried about your silence... I am in the seventh
month and very tense...*

I hug you

Ines

Rita my dear,

*... Today's paper says that the troubles are not over yet in
Palestine and Jews are defending themselves. I have a friend
named Leon Moshe who has been in Palestine for over a year and
says that this situation cannot continue...*

*Your brother,
Semiko*

On June 17th, Ines' eldest son, Solomon, writes to Rita telling her of the
birth of his new sister, Rachelle, as well as reminding them of Salonica's new
name, Thessaloniki.[59]

Dear Aunt Rita and Uncle Sam,

*... We received your precious letter with the beautiful pictures...
Are the children all healthy? Uncle Sam looks very skinny, what's
the reason?... The good news is that we became three Matarassos
with the birth of Rachelle who is so beautiful... Mother gave birth
so fast... Within three hours, the contractions began and by eight
o'clock we became three...Don't be sad that Mama gave birth to a
daughter and not a boy that can be named after Uncle Benjamin...
there is already a Benjamin in Uncle Leon's family...The doctor
ordered Mom to rest in bed for 15 days... Mom asks if it's possible
for you to write to Uncle Isaac for her.... I have been very busy
with the exams. I will finish school in three years and then go to
work to help my dear father...*

Solomon

P.S.

*In all the letters you write from now on, you must write
Thessaloniki and not Salonica, because this is the official name of
the city, by law, otherwise the letter will not arrive.*

The drama of Sami's engagement begins and is announced in August by a
string of letters, both to Rita and Leon.

Dear Rita,

*I have good news for you, I got engaged to a girl, Rachelle,
the daughter of a tailor-dealer, Mr. Aaron Levy. He has three
daughters; the two older ones are already married... She is a
good, quiet and honest girl who has always lived a decent life, her
father is a well-known and respected tailor and was educated in the
Italian school... The more I know her, the more I like her...*

Sam

My dear Rita,

*... I take care of the baby with the help of my mother-in-law...I
continue to work to meet the many expenses of the house...Moise
feels better, but is still very thin and always tired...*

*I want to tell you about Semico's engagement. Two years ago
he wanted to get married but I tried to get it out of his mind
because he was still too young and anyway it was Elico's turn...
but now an opportunity arose with Rachelle Levy whom we did
not know. I since heard good things about her. I then spoke
to his brothers and since at the moment they did not intend to
marry, there would be no reason to delay Semico. On Saturday,
a visit was made to the bride's house. She lives next door to Dr.
Menasche's house, and we were all invited to eat. It was a very
happy occasion...*

*... Five days ago I went up to Benjamin's and Dad's graves, on my
own because Mom can't come. I brought them candies to celebrate
Sam's engagement and prayed a lot for everyone... Alegré no
longer goes to Benjamin's grave. She "came out" of mourning and
when she came to Mom once in six months, it was just to upset her
or to ask for money... [Figure 36].*

Ines

Dear Rita,

*... Dino and I gave up our place in the queue to Sami with great
pleasure...You know that we don't pay attention to what people
say. The girl looks very pleasant... She finds her place quickly,
and knows how to respond well, she is well-educated and perfectly
fluent in French and Italian...the engagement is next week and
the wedding three months later, I hope you do not miss the event...
Don't worry Rita, my turn will be coming soon. About Dino, he has*

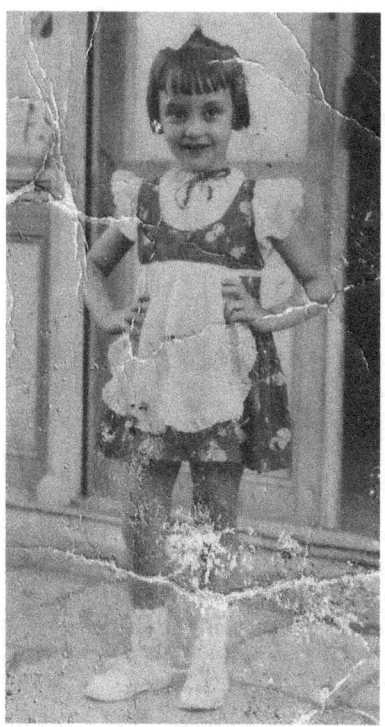

Figure 36 Benjamin's Rachelle.

no intention yet...Recently, we received a letter from Dear Leon asking for your address...How is your Sam's business? He should probably know Yiddish and Arabic well by now because he trades with Poles and Arabs.[60]

Eli

Leon is, of course, kept in the loop too and is sent letters by Ines, Eli and Sam, with the odd line from Dino and Henri to announce the good news of Sam's engagement. He is now in a position to send money to his family, which goes mainly towards the medical expenses for his mother...

Dear Leon,

... I think about all the excitement of these days and I do not know how to begin, I am glad, very happy that something happened to me that I longed for. Since I became engaged I feel completely connected with my fiancée, new feelings are born in me, new and

*sweet feelings that I had never experienced before... I do not
know if these things should be written on paper, but I think that a
brother is like a neighbour in another body...*

*But for our dear Isaac, a brother is a man who happened to be born
overweight and without any further importance... I may be wrong,
and I would love to know that I was wrong about him... this is how
I am, I can't help saying what I am thinking...*

Sami

Dear Leon,

*... Mom thanks you very much for your beautiful words....She
suffers from high blood pressure and must see the doctor often.
She also gets knee injections, which costs a lot, and sometimes
she can't pay, so the money you sent is a great blessing... She
wanted to write a few words, but for now she can't ... I talked to
Moise about the money you want to send us to Mom, he suggested
sending through the Ottoman bank in Paris... If you are thinking
of sending money by mail, please do so by registered mail with the
stated amount to...*

Ines

Sam appears from these letters as having a poetic streak. His letters express
so much joy at the engagement in August, so when it is called off in December, it is heart-wrenching.

Dear Leon,

*... I know that you've been waiting for this letter for a long time...
we were busy with all the marriage arrangements. Thinking about
the best date and worrying about the honeymoon etc. But then...
at the end of November, the director of the company I work for
came and said that one of the workers needs to be sacked. And
so, as I was the last one to have been taken, it was me who had to
be sent home... This was a bomb for me and my wedding plans,
and of course for my fiancée and her family. The wedding was
postponed because I didn't think I could get married when I was
unemployed... Ines' husband Moise found a job for me a few days
later in a rubber factory as a bookkeeper, but the salary was two-
thirds of what I was earning, but I had to take it, it is better than
to risk remaining unemployed at this time...So you will understand
why I was late in responding to your letter. In the meantime, I*

*can't get married until I find a better job... otherwise, everything
is fine... Mom has become old suddenly. She complains about
the cold and how much she misses you... My fiancée was very
disappointed and sad as everything was ready for the wedding and
now we had to postpone it.... I hope everything will work out for
the better soon...*

Sami

1938 – Rachelle Cohen dies

Marie Bonaparte, Napoleon's great-grandniece, saved Sigmund Freud and members of his family by paying for their escape route from Vienna to London in 1938. She was married to Prince George (1869–1957), the second son of the Greek King George I (1845–1913).[61] In 1938, she lived in Paris, not far away from Leon Cohen, during the same years. But there's another Jewish family that her family saved in those years.

Marie's sister-in-law Alice, or Princess Andrew as was her title, suffered a mental breakdown and was later diagnosed with schizophrenia. Freud himself was consulted and diagnosed her, without seeing her, as suffering from sexual frustration. He recommended in 1930 "X-raying her ovaries in order to kill off her libido".[62]

Alice herself had to deal with a complicated reality: her only son Philip fought on the British side during World War II, while her two sons-in-law fought on the Nazi side. She herself was living in Athens during the war, separated from her husband, who held clear Nazi sympathies. She lived with her brother-in-law George and Marie in their big three-storey house at the centre of the city. She was active in the Red Cross and organized soup kitchens and shelters for orphans with the help of her sister Louise Alexandra Marie Irene Mountbatten (1889–1965), who was married to Gustaf VI Adolf (1882–1973), King of Sweden, and flew often to Sweden to bring supplies.

When the Italians were defeated in 1943, the Nazi forces occupied the city, and the Jewish population feared the same fate that their brethren in Salonica had suffered. Many of them did.

Alice was approached by a widowed Rachelle Cohen and two of her five children, Tilde and Michel (the other three escaped to Egypt and joined the exile Greek Government there), and sought refuge. Alice remained true to a promise made by her father-in-law, King George I, in 1913, when Rachel's husband, Haimaki Cohen, aided him. She and Prince Nicholas, her brother-in-law, were the only remaining members of the royal family in Athens, and they sheltered the Cohens until the end of the war. For that, she was awarded by Yad Vashem "Righteous Among the Nations" in 1994 in a ceremony in Jerusalem when her son Philip was present.

Even though she died in Buckingham Palace, she had made a wish that was honoured with some reservations on the part of her family, and her remains were transferred to the Convent of Saint Mary Magdalene in Gethsemane on the Mount of Olives in Jerusalem (near her aunt Grand Duchess Elizabeth Feodorovna, a Russian Orthodox saint) in 1988, nearly two decades after her death in 1969.

In June 2018, her great-grandson, Prince William (b. 1982), made the first-ever official British Royal visit to Israel, where, amongst other things, he visited her grave as well as meeting Rachel Cohen's descendants, Edith and Phillipe Cohen.

So, one Rachelle Cohen and her family survived in Athens through the aid of the Greek Royal family. It was not "my" Rachelle Cohen...

The year 1938 belongs to her. It was perhaps the hardest year before the curtain fell on the Cohens in Salonica and Paris. The year began with the reports of the deteriorating health of Rachelle.

The letters from Salonica to Paris and Tel-Aviv during 1938 ran along parallel lines. Ines and her brothers made sure to update Leon and Rita on a regular basis, often complaining about not receiving enough letters from them. It seemed that the Salonica branch had a greater need to keep in touch with the outposts. Many of the letters carried similar messages.

February

Dear Rita,

... I can imagine how difficult it is with 3 children to sit down and write a letter home... I was glad to read that you take better care of your teeth... Mom had the flu but is better now. I go and take care of her every day, leaving my own children alone...

Ines

March

Dear Leon,

We haven't heard from you in 3 months and we're worried. Sam has written to you twice and received no reply... Ines is very happy with her cute girl who starts to smile and make cute movements and we spend hours with her.

Little Benjamin, how is he? Has he started talking? In the picture he looks a little naughty... [Figure 37].

Yours,
Eli

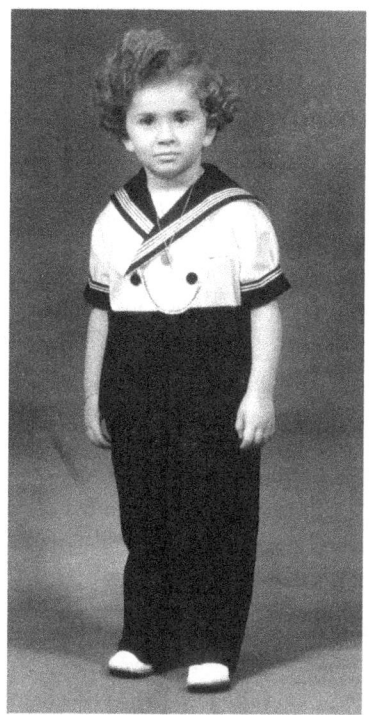

Figure 37 Benjamin Cohen.

April

Leon dear,

I can't underst and why you do not write... Mom is getting very old and can't be disturbed. She waits for your letters and she doesn't fall asleep at night. And we don't know what to think either. I hope you have no serious reason except lack of time. How do you feel? How is the health and business? Is your wife okay? Benjamin? My hands tremble as I write my brother's name, this holy man... I've had two nasal surgeries recently. They helped me a lot with the difficulties I was having breathing... today I am almost fine, and hope all problems will soon disappear... I did not suffer from pain (the most painful moment was paying the doctor)...

Sami

May

Dear Rita,

*Why so quiet? I wait impatiently every day for a letter from you...
I have a lot of daily worries having to look after our old and sick
mother whose nostalgia for her children abroad makes her more
and more sick... Leon too does not write... I wrote to him many
times without getting an answer, and all this causes great grief to
our good mother who is also so full of sorrow after our Benjamin's
death.... My Solomon has been ill for 15 days with scarlatina, he
has to stay home for 40 days, during which time Nelly went to stay
with my sister-in-law... I am sending a picture taken by an amateur
photographer... it is so small I am doubtful that you will be able to
recognize us... [Figure 38].*

Ines

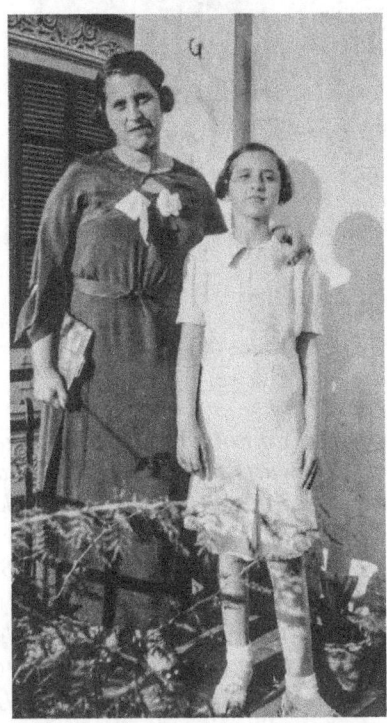

Figure 38 Ines and Nelly Matarasso.

August

My dear brother Leon,

… In my last letter, I wrote to you that I was fired from my job at Mario Salmon because of a lack of business…I was then employed in a rubber products factory, where I earn 1500 drachmas a month. I managed to get a job with Henry Angel at 2250 drachmas a month, it's not huge but I manage to get along… My fiancée's family have not been very warm towards me after the loss of my previous job. My future mother-in-law met me one day and wanted to cancel the engagement. Believe me, this has caused me a great deal of suffering…

Sami

September

Dear Leon,

I write to you to tell you about Mother's illness. We cannot cure her, because her illness is hopeless…Isaac was reluctant to reply to my letters. This happens when you are not rich… He forgets all that I did for him when he was in school…My brother-in-law will go to Marseille to see his parents and can deliver a package to you, but he won't be able to get to Paris, so Mr. Aaron Avagon might be the go-between…He will leave Thessaloniki next week… you should go look for him… Do you have used clothes like shirts? Ask Isaac too, you can give it to my brother-in-law Isidore Crispin when he returns to Thessaloniki, they're for my kids.

Ines

October

Dear Rita and Sam,

I am very concerned that I did not receive any reply to my last … I'm sure you're going through difficult times now, you have no idea how much we worry… Several of our friends are arriving in Palestine soon…Sarah, her neighbour, Rebecca Cohen, a sister of Leon and Abraham Rekanti, so please welcome them because they are my good neighbours. She'll give you a box of Tejos (Sweets) and some Quaramelas for the girls… tell your kids that "These are Aunt Ines who is dying from longing for you…" We have just

received a letter from Dear Leon and Bondy and they say that
Bondy is pregnant again!

I hug you and love you.

Your sister,
Ines

November

Dear Leon,

... It is important to bring Mom good news because she is
constantly in pain... I was glad to hear that Bondy is pregnant
again.... Mom asks you to send more elastic stockings for her
veins. If you see Isaac and even if you don't, you must know that
we are all very angry, why did he forget about us? What did we do
to him?

Ines

December 3rd arrives with the news of Rachelle's death. They all write
to Rita and Leon on a special paper, which is framed with black mourning lines, each repeating the details of Rachelle's last days. The letters are
brought in sequence, a testimony of their pain as if read over her open grave.

... With tears in my eyes I am writing to you... we are without our
dear mother... can you imagine that eight days ago we went to the
confectionery store together ...On Tuesday, she got the flu and the
doctor used cupping glasses to help her... but two days later she got
angina and a cardiologic complication developed...We called for
the doctors who were with her but we were not lucky enough.... It
only got worse...

I was very lonely and in great distress. She died in Moise's arms
because I stayed with the boys at home...

Ines

...You're probably expecting a letter from us....It's really hard to
write to you about dear mother's passing... now, after a whole week
has gone by, we are still confused in an unspeakable way...What
can we say about our mother's death?... You can be sure, that we
have done all we could to keep her alive but she had incurable
diseases.

Sami

... We are still under the cruel blow that landed on us... our good
and revered mother that we would no longer be able to see... her

life has been one great sacrifice for her children. I don't want to make you sad, but my heart melts as I write these bitter words to you, we must comfort each other because of the blow we received... Since 14.11.38 she did not feel well, and despite all the medical treatment it got worse...the doctor said that her heart was very weak, and immediately we consulted with three cardiologists who said she had developed angina of her chest. We took a nurse who was with her day and night, but to no avail, on November 17th, her condition got even worse, and another consultation was made with three doctors who said there was nothing to do and that science in this case could not help... With her last breath and last kisses, she returned her soul on Friday, November 18, at 9:30 am. At four thirty in the morning, she was still laughing with the nurse, who understood what was about to happen and laughed with tears in her eyes. She treated her with dedication as if she were her daughter... this blow will not be forgotten and we will cry all our lives... Mother was buried near Benjamin...the expenses are huge and we thank you, Leon, for helping us with the expenses of pharmacies, doctors, funeral taxes, all amounting to more than 15000 drachmas which we still owe...

Eli

... I don't know how to start this bitter letter, a sad moment for me to tell you how in just a few days we lost our dear and beloved mother... we did not see it coming...she sacrificed her life for us and was an example of mother and wife, educated us, guided us, fed us in our sickness, and sacrificed her health for us.

Kiss the kids for me.

Your brother with tears in his eyes,
Henri

Nobody knows exactly how old Rachelle Cohen was when she died. Her birth certificate was burnt in the fire that consumed many public records in Salonica in 1917. Perhaps, she was in her eighties, perhaps younger. She was not a healthy woman for most of her adult life, and the last years, which were characterized with emotional agony and physical hardships, did not help. Widowed in her forties, she carried the burden of raising her children on her own with dignity. A family story describes that when there was not enough food on the table during the hard years, she drew the curtains lest people could see their destitution. She also insisted on wearing white gloves when she went outside, maintaining appearances. Her death, painful as it was, at least saved her from the terrible years that were to follow and the gruesome deaths her children and grandchildren suffered in Auschwitz.

1939 – Bereavement

On May 29th, Hannah Arendt, on her way to her safe haven in the USA wrote from Paris to her German-born colleague, Gershom Scholem (1897–1982), the philosopher and historian in Palestine, where he had been living since 1923. She was staying in the 14th arrondissement, a mere 4 kms from Leon and Bondy's flat. She wrote of the plights of the Jews in Paris. A year later, in another letter to Scholem, this time from the south of France, she writes that Jews are dying in Europe and are found lying in the fields. In the very same letter, she announces the suicide of their mutual friend, the German philosopher Walter Benjamin (1892–1940), on the French–Spanish border, on his own escape route to the U.S.A., as he feared that the Spaniards would not let him enter the country.

In France, a few months before the government declared war on Nazi Germany in September, along with the UK, a film was released in June. *Le Jour Se Lève* (The Day Breaks), based upon a script by Jacques Prévert (1900–1977) and directed by Marcel Carné (1906–1996), it showed the story of a young man, played by Jean Gabin (1904–1976), barracked in his room after he had shot a man with whom his lover was having an affair. It was released and shown in Paris, soon to be besieged by the Nazis, until the Vichy government banned it.[63] Did Leon and Bondy see the film? Did they have the peace of mind that would have allowed them to go out? Could they get a babysitter to watch over little Benjamin?

The family in Salonica is trying to recover from Rachelle's death. Leon is in a position to help, as the string of letters from Salonica show...

January

My dear Leon,

... We thank you for your prompt response in helping us pay our debt for our late mother, this shows how committed you are to your family... not comparing this to anyone else... You must believe that we did our best to keep Mom alive, but she got worse very fast and the doctors did their best in those difficult moments. Her

death was very difficult, and I still cannot be convinced that she is gone. I feel her presence at home and keep expecting to see her. I dreamt about her at night many times and then sit and cry like a little child... she was a good mother and a model for a beloved and devoted mother.... I hope dear Leon that you are in good health and dear Bondy will soon give birth without much pain...

Hugging you

Yours,
Sami

February

My dear brother,

... You are right to be surprised to receive news from me, as they are so rare that you only expect news from Eli, Sami and Ines... I'm a little busier than them, so I leave the letter writing to them... it is pointless to repeat things that others have already written to you, about the meaning of Mother's passing for all of us. This disaster cannot be compared to anything else. The pen cannot express what one feels. For me, it was a big shock and emptiness... now that we have lost the woman of the family, it is more difficult for us to start our own families... As for Binyaminico – give him a big kiss so he knows it came from a man who is very far away... Ines wrote to Isaac, hoping we would hear from him soon. It's sad not to receive a letter from my brother in such a situation. Why doesn't he write? Is he angry with us? And if so, what did we do to deserve this? Henri rarely writes to you...he does not want to communicate about how he is, unlucky and has no job, and nobody outside the family is willing to help him. We do our best to help him...

Kissing
Dino

March

...We got the joyous news of Leon's and Body's Rachelle's birth -27.2.39 [Figure 39]. It is good to have some joy in the family after the departure of the dear mother. Last Sunday we went to her grave....

Eli

...Our poor mother would have been so happy with the news.... She wanted to come and see you, she always said that when she learned that Bondy was pregnant again... Rita is also 7 months pregnant for the fourth time and having quite a hard time...[64] *I wrote to*

Isaac as you asked...I explained we were very worried by his long silence after the sad news of our dear mother's death. If you see him ask him why he doesn't answer...It is very sad to be forgotten by one of your brothers...And what does Benimino say? Does he love his sister or is he already jealous of her?

Ines

May

To my dear brother Leon,

... It is true that I rarely write...but you know I am not the same Henri who used to joke and laugh because the burden of supporting a large family leads you to change your character... I thank you for your willingness to come to my aid...How is Bondy? How is Benjamin? Is he as stubborn as we are, as we all were?...Thanks so much for the cheque which I cashed already....

Henri

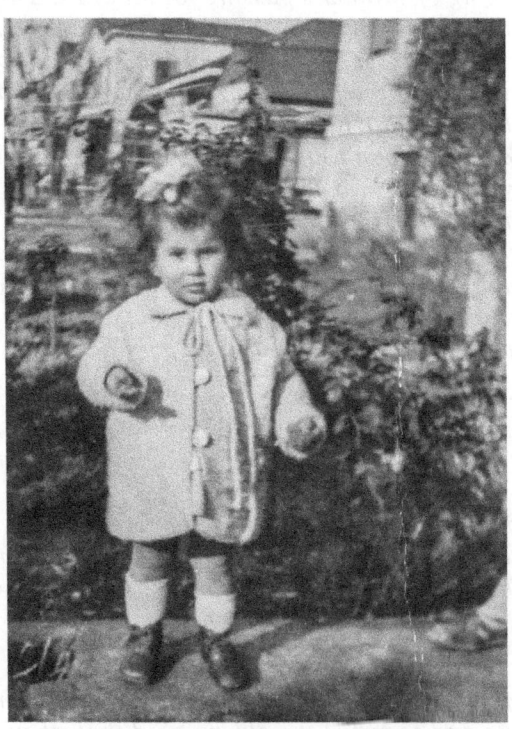

Figure 39 Leon's and Body's Rachelle Cohen.

In May Leon writes both to his family in Salonica and his sister in Tel-Aviv. He types both letters and keeps a carbon copy. A sense of history?

Dear Ines,

... You need to know that times have changed...Unfortunately, I am not in a good economic situation and that of Isaac is no better... I am sorry I cannot help more with Henri.... I have sent a cheque in his name for 500 francs... I cannot do more because, as you know, having two young children incurs many expenses....I believe that because I am doing well at work and thanks to Bondy who knows how to manage the house properly, we hope to able to see the light at the end of the tunnel soon...We would love to hear from you and your children, Solomon, Nelly and Rachelle ...

I find it difficult to accept that mother is no longer with us...I sincerely hope that political events will calm down and that we will not have the incessant threat of war, which makes it hard for us to know which way to turn not knowing where to go... Maybe when the threat passes and with some luck, we can go to Thessaloniki and see you and pray on the graves of our loved ones...Our little Elliane Reschelika is two months old now. Thanks to Bondy's dedicated care, she is perfectly healthy. Our little Benjamin, he is a naughty little demon, he brings us all joy, but a fair amount of work for Bondy.

In Paris it is very difficult to raise children...

> *Rachelle, Benjamin, Bondy and Leon*

Dear Rita,

We are pleased to inform you of the birth of our Elliane (Reschelika) who was born on February 27, 1939 at 4 AM

The baby is well. Although the days prior to birth were very difficult for Bondy, she received help and support and the birth itself passed quickly and well with tears of joy.... Now, she is named after our mother as her birth came after our mother's death in the same way that Benjamin's birth came after our brother's death... I miss hearing from you... Your kids must be big already. Who knows maybe someday we'll have the opportunity to meet, maybe in Paris or maybe in Palestine...

> *Leon and Bondy*

On a parallel and almost identical path, the letters to Rita in Palestine are a chronicle of sadness.

January

Darling Sam and Rita,

... With tears in my eyes I answer your dear letter... we mourn the death of our mother and cry with our brothers who were left alone...I was very moved to read that you are pregnant again. Was this what was missing for you? It is all so exhausting...But we have no choice, we are mothers of families and we have to look after our sons and husbands... Rita, my soul, I'm very alone. My highlight of the week was to go to Mom every Saturday and now I have nowhere to go... Cry Rita, cry for mother and Benjamin, but don't let yourself be sick of it. I part with tears in my eyes...

Ines

March

Rita my dear,

...I write a few lines to tell you that I am very worried about your long silence...

I do not fall asleep in bed, thinking maybe you are sick and maybe the children are not well... I am alone, completely alone and I do not see anyone. I only go out to see the dentist... for quite a while I was toothless but now I have dentures so I can eat again...

Poor mother was very upset when she saw me toothless...On Sunday, we were out visiting the graves of Mom, Benjamin and Dad in the cemetery... My sister, I want to be near you, see you and take comfort from my sister, to hold you and cry together... What to do that we are separated and maybe for life, I miss you so much...

Ines

April

Dear Rita,

... On the first night of Passover, I invited everybody here and we all read the Haggadah together... I try to take care of them as much as I can... they find a home here, and I take care of them in

*every way... Thank you so much my dear little sister for the socks,
I really liked them... Isaac has not answered me to this day, what
to do, this is life. We are very worried about him, he may have
problems with his wife...If you have a boy, we think he should be
called Benjamin since Dad's name is "already" with Henri.*

I hug you tight

Ines

May

Dear Rita,

*... we were very happy to hear about the birth of the twins, but
we are also worried about the extra financial burden that will be
for you. But I am sure God will not forget Sam and he will have
a flourishing business so that he can fulfill his commitment as a
father and raise his children according to his heart's desire.*

*I know Sam pretty well and I appreciate his persistence. He can
always count on our support – within our means – as if he were our
blood brother.*

*I hope you recover your strength soon as you now have to care for
two more babies.*

Eli and Dino

And Isaac? The subject of so much worry and angst surfaces after a long
absence and seemingly is oblivious to all these tidings, continuing along the
same track as this letter of February 21st shows

Dear Leon,

*... You'll probably be surprised to get news from me... I am now
preparing for the International Fair in (unclear)... Good business
but there are many expenses for the hotel and the like. I am
currently having difficulties and I need your help.*

*You know that if I ask for your help, it's a sign that I'm in trouble
that I couldn't know beforehand. I am ready to deposit Martha's
jewelry in exchange for 1500 to 2000 francs which I urgently need.
It is worth ten times more. There are a pair of platinum earrings, a
single diamond, etc., it's worth much more, but I don't trust anyone
but you. I pledge to repay you as soon as my work in the north*

ends. I mean in early May and maybe even earlier. Because the fair begins on the first of May.

I do not think you will refuse me and I urge you to urgently set a date to meet because I need to return immediately.

Kisses to Bondy and Benjamin and I would love to hear about the event you are looking forward to.

Your brother,
Isaac

And for the first time recorded, Leon answers back, angrily. This is Leon's seventeenth letter in the collection, and also the last one, until the two letters he sent from Drancy.

My dear brother,

Your letter made me very sad... What makes you think I have 1500 to 2000 francs to spare? And even if I did, what can I do with Martha's jewelry? Guarantee? Do you think I'm a loan shark? You know that Mother passed away and you didn't think it was your duty to write home. I'm not accusing you of anything but you can't make any claims on me either...We expect Bondy to give birth any day now. She is in a maternity ward which is quite costly. I may have to borrow money myself... You came at a bad time. I'm just sorry you didn't think about it before...

A long silence but again, in September, Isaac carries on desperately, evoking all that he can to get Leon to help him. It is the cry of a desperate man, perhaps his last cry for help. It is the last recorded exchange between the two brothers that we have on record. Was Leon able to help him? Was the sense of urgency and danger in Isaac's letter genuine or was it yet again one of his ploys?

Dear Leon,

...Martha phoned your wife's parents because she wanted to see you urgently. You must, I repeat must help me urgently with the 1000 francs I need today. I have almost 4,000 francs in receipt of valuables which I deposited that I offer to you as a guarantee... I ask you not only as a brother, but as the person Martha and I received with open arms and without thinking twice when you arrived in France... You must remember our years together and

you must come to my aid today... Leon, I understand that you cannot raise such a sum alone, but you can ask your father-in-law to help... It's very serious, now more than ever... We will be waiting for you at home tomorrow evening. We are at the Legendre Cinema on 3rd Legendary Street every night. We will be there from 0730 to 0930 or later at home. I need your answer by 10 o'clock at the very latest.

Leon, you must hurry, you must...In memory of our dear mother and dear father, help me, save me.

Your brother
Isaac

The last item in 1939 is a letter from Sami in September, a dark, threatening letter.

Dear Leon,

... we are all waiting for a letter from you... we do not know if you are recruited, and how is Isaac... write to us as quickly as possible...we are concerned about you... none of us was recruited yet. I hope we will be able to continue our correspondence...

Your brother
Sami

What happened in the next couple of years is almost too terrible to tell. It has become a cliché to say that the horrors of the Holocaust cannot be retold with language. And yet, these words must be written down. I find I have less and less to say as the postmemory progresses. It develops and dissolves at the same time, like so much water, I try to cup with my mental hands and hold the precious few last drops of evidence of these last three years.

1940 – The family saga

The Nazis arrived in Paris in June 1940. The Cohens and Saüls were deported from Paris on November 11th 1942. What was left of Paris was liberated from the Nazis in August 1943.

Only four letters are left from 1940, two to Rita and two to Leon. It is futile to wonder why they wrote so little. In fact, it is a wonder they wrote at all, realising what conditions they were living under. The few details they provide are enough to paint the grim picture. The knowledge of what's to come makes it even grimmer. It is amazing to read how important family ties remain for them in Salonica, Paris and Tel-Aviv. Those invisible strings create a network that seems to be throbbing with longing and love. They share all kinds of details about their lives, trying to incorporate the siblings into their lives, trying to fill the distance with life.

In January, Isaac, still on the run, still hustling writes to Leon.

Leon dear,

I got your letter... can we meet in Paris? Passing through Pramantans Cafe on 60 Rue Lafayette at about 3 or 6 o'clock...I am glad to know that you all feel well...

Kiss Bondy and my nephews from Martha and me...

> *Salud*
> *Isaac*

On February 27th, Dino writes to Leon. This is the very last letter that was sent to Leon that exists.

Dear Leon,

Please send us a picture of Rachelle whom we do not know and kiss her on our behalf.... A few words from Bondy will make us

*very happy, I know she is very busy with the children, but only a
few words. I imagine Benjamin is a serious little man and not a
bad guy at home, and that he wants to know his uncles who are
far away and who never come to see him. That's not fair on our
part but what to do? Here we are all fine, except for the insanity...
Henri is now working as a coal salesman and he makes a living.
My business is thriving and I hope yours will too, during the war...*

*Kisses to everyone from me and don't forget our dear Isaac and
Uncle Albert.*

Your brother who loves you
Dino

On March 28th, Ines writes

Dear Rita,

*Why are you not answering my letters? How can I understand this
long silence?*

Are you sick? Or does the weather cause you problems as it does to me?

*You probably know that winter here is very hard and long. Big
snowflakes dropped yesterday and today it's very cold. If I
neglected you for so long, it was because I was twice ill with the
flu. I had to be in bed for three weeks doing a serious diet following
the urine test...My mother-in-law was ill almost all winter long.
Bronchitis along with pneumonia. You can imagine, my dear sister,
what we have been through. I was so tired from helping her that
I myself fell sick. Today, I have to take a maid because I can no
longer work and because doctors have forbidden me to work... How
many times I have talked to you in my head during my illness, dear
Rita, I was alone... In the past our dear mother came to visit me.
I miss and always think of her...The affection of my children does
not satisfy me... but we have to accept it and remember better
times...*

And on October 29th, her son Solomon writes

Dear Aunt Rita,

*I have the honour to write to you that we all feel good...Uncle Eli
is currently staying with us, after closing their house. Answer us
quickly...*

Your nephew
Solomon

When telling my relatives about my interest in the family letters and trying to write about the family's experience, I would often hear very mixed reactions, ranging from deep appreciation of my efforts to sheer puzzlement as to why I was still so preoccupied with these past events.

The ambivalence was perhaps due to the fact that they could not tolerate the pain and guilt evoked in them by the knowledge that those stories were there to be told but they were not able, nor willing, to hear them. They were children when their mother plied them with the stories. They wanted to live differently, they wanted to build the State of Israel and be strong and healthy Israelis, Sabras, and not bear the guilt of the survivors, not to be branded with the scars of the testimony to the pain that was left behind but was present in their mother's eyes.

Their reluctance and denial was not unique amongst their generation. As Wardi (1992) recounted in her book upon second-generation Holocaust survivors, dealing with the unspeakable trauma was an emotional burden many individuals could not face directly. The sense of family catastrophe was so intense and reached so deep into their sense of security that their only way of protecting themselves from the traumatic impact was by denying its relevance to them. In a sense, the postmemory had to jump a generation in order to be registered in any intelligible and communicable form.

Their generation, the second generation of Holocaust survivors, often chose not to listen, not to remember. But that conscious decision did not prevent a single iota of traumatic material from seeping deep under their skin, directly into the core of their being, filling up every available hole in their soul.

It took many years for all that toxic material to evolve within them and then explode. Small explosions, at the beginning. Then another, then another, till the chain reaction was devastating, leaving no stone unturned.

Each of Rita's and Shmuel's children had his or her turn of being in the middle of the explosion, either as the explosive material or the victim of the explosion. Nobody was spared.

It is nobody's fault. The way they reacted to Rita's pain is perhaps unique to them, but many families in Israel bear the terrible hallmark of being second-generation Holocaust survivors. Each wound is unique, but all are caused by the same kind of toxic material.

None of Rita's five children is pathological in nature. All are quite normal. All have settled into a routine family life. All have married well and raised healthy and functioning children. All are working people and form a part of the lively and flourishing Israeli society. When meeting at family occasions such as Friday night gatherings, Bar Mitzvahs, weddings and the like, all seem to be happy. Also, they all seem to like one another. But, as any of their adult children will tell you, things are not as they seem.

Over the last thirty years, since both their parents have died in old age, friction has been one of the dominant sounds in their relationships. Over that period, there has always been at least one of the five siblings who was not on speaking terms with the others, or some of the others. The overt cause of such falling-out had been mostly minor events, such as not returning calls or responding in an offensive matter. There were no big issues at stake, no financial issues. Their parents did not leave behind much property and what was left was divided equally amongst the siblings. The disputed inheritance was not earthly materials.

Friction of course exists in all families. Most families manage to control areas of discord by normal defensive and avoidance behaviours that allow that friction to remain under the surface without disrupting their lives.

When did it all begin? Hard to say. It is clear to me that the friction became toxic over the handling of the letters, once they were discovered and read. But there were warning signs of the powerful undercurrents years before, even before the elders were dead.

Perhaps one place, of the many possible knots, to start unravelling the entanglement is the story of the marriage of Benjamin Parenti, one of the twins Rita gave birth to in 1939.[65] He married an American Jew whom he had met while studying and living in the USA during the 1970s. When the young couple returned to Israel with the plan of setting up a home there, the family reception towards the bride was at best lukewarm. Most of the time, she was the target of supposedly humorous verbal cantering. Being from a different cultural background and of a gentle emotional disposition, she was perceived to be very different from the rest of the family.

Her poor reception by the family was not an unusual occurrence in Israel in those days and her story does reflect a certain prejudice that existed, and still does, between the Ashkenazi and Sephardim Jewish communities. The rift between her husband and the rest of the family was a result of those early days. Though they did settle in Israel and started a thriving family including two lovely children, the scars of those early days did not heal completely and once their children had left home, Benjamin turned against his brother and sisters and accused them of cruelty towards his wife. Those accusations resulted in a break-up between him and his siblings which was accompanied by acrimonious verbal exchanges, some of which were conducted though emails and a family internet forum that was formed to enable contact with some of the family members who had moved abroad.

His estrangement from the family lasted a couple of years and began a series of other estrangements between different siblings. Each of the siblings took turns at acting the role of the injured party, often with some justice. From their point of view, the injury inflicted was always huge. To a bystander, or even to the children of the siblings, it appeared almost comical. It was clear that the siblings were taking turns without being aware of it. Even after they were made aware, the acrimonious episode had to run its full, convoluted course, sometimes lasting many months. Each, in turn, was also eventually reconciled with the rest of the siblings, usually during some family occasions and with the pretext that the reconciliation and the forgiving was a generous sacrifice made for the benefit of the rest.

Benjamin himself had already died, as did the husbands of two of the sisters. The current status is relatively quiet. The remaining siblings are all in their eighties, some healthier than others. Their days together are numbered. The wounds are perhaps no longer bleeding but the scars are still visible. The toxicity has perhaps been exhausted by old age.

The relevance of the letters of the Cohens, not so unique in itself, to this family drama became evident over the handling of the actual letters over the last twenty years, since they were revealed. The questions as to who the guardian will be, the rightful keeper of the boxes of letters, in whose house would they be held, became a toxic issue. Countless arguments, accusations and counteraccusations were exchanged. Not all siblings showed the same passionate interest in the holding of this treasure, Benjamin himself was already dead, but the dispute was passionately shared by them all. It was suggested by more than one grandchildren (themselves all adults with families of their own by now), who witnessed these exchanges with a mixture of amusement, shame and horror, that it was as if the siblings were arguing over the possession of the letters as if they were the actual remains of the parents themselves. It was only finally practically resolved when an agreement was reached to hand over the contents of the four boxes to Yad Vashem, as recounted earlier in the book. So, today, the physical remains are no longer in any of the siblings' possessions, but the hurt is still there. Perhaps, never to heal. Perhaps, some wounds can never truly heal. Perhaps, some memories can never be left alone.

One current consolation is that the next generation, my generation, seems to be able to contain and put a stop to the toxic passing on of these materials. To date, no real tensions have shown themselves. Perhaps, they have been buried and truly mourned never to re-emerge. Or perhaps, the time will come that the toxicity will show itself again?

1941 – The silence deepens

Greece's involvement in World War II began on October 28th 1940 with the irruption of a predatory Italian force across the Albanian border. After fierce fighting in harsh winter conditions, a Greek army, which included 13,000 Jewish soldiers, drove them back. Italian failure brought a swift reaction.

On April 9th 1941, Salonica became the first Greek city to be seized by Wehrmacht forces. Greece was divided between Germany, Italy and Bulgaria. Salonica, as a part of Macedonia, fell under German rule.[66] Greece overall was secondary in Hitler's big plan and the tripartite division reflected that. Therefore, the implementation of the Nuremberg racial laws took longer, as the Nazis found it hard to coax their Bulgarian and Italian partners to cooperate. The Nazis began by anti-Semitic steps in Salonica: requisition and billeting, closing the local Jewish newspaper, *Messagero,* and arresting political figures.

In Tel-Aviv, Rita Cohen sits at home, already mother of five, wondering what had become of her family.

On February 12th, Ines writes to Rita. This is the very last letter from Salonica.

Rita my darling,

Why this long silence? Are you sick, dear? Why don't you give us any good news? I received a letter from (unclear) *in which he tells me "Rita and the kids feel good" but it is not enough, dear Rita, you have to write at least one word. Everything is going well with us, and we are still waiting for better days... Dino and Sam write often and feel good.[67] Eli has been living with us for three months. You do not have to worry, we are well protected from the streets...*
            Kiss the little ones, write to us quickly.

Rita indeed responded quickly and sent a letter that never reached its destination and was returned to her. Did she then begin to fear and perhaps realize what was beginning to happen?

Dear Brothers, dear Sister,

I am replying again to your last letter. I sent you a small photo in the last letter. I hope you received it. How are you all feeling? Please write regularly. I want to read.... (unclear words). I have not heard from you for three months. Why isn't Eli writing? Or Henri?

We are safe. God is watching us and may look after us all. We kiss you and hope to hear from you soon.

Rita and Sam

There are no more letters in the boxes. They are empty. It is time to start the end of this postmemory. To return home. To the present. But not quite yet. Returning home is not so simple when you know it is a home besieged with loss such as this. Perhaps, it is better to linger a bit more along the way, whistling in the dark. Some details still need to be remembered and ironed out before I can lay this postmemory to rest.

So, is the story complete? Can it ever be?

1942 – The last days: Drancy

1942. The boxes are empty. This is the skeletal end.

Of what happened to Leon and his family after the boxes have been exhausted we only know through the letters which were sent by various members of the Saül family, including Leon and Bondy from the Drancy internment camp. These letters were kept by the Saül family after the war. They need hardly any explanation.

Drancy is a suburb of Paris, located about 11 kms north-east of the city centre. It was initially built as a modern urban complex. It was used by the French Vichy regime police, and later the Nazi SS force, as an internment and detention centre between June 22nd 1942 and July 31st 1944, for about 67,000 French, German and Polish Jews who were deported to the death camps in sixty-four rail convoys during that period. Only about 1,500 people survived the Drancy camp or the concentration camps they were sent to.[68]

The first member of the family to be taken to Drancy was Michel (July 20th or 21st 1941 – there had been a general roundup of young Salonician men). The rest arrived in the camp in the first week of November, and then they all left on November 11th. These letters, also kept by Rosa, are the only testimony to the time they spent in Drancy.

Michel Saül to his parents Drancy, November 1st, 1942

My dear parents, dear everyone,

I have received your letter from October the 18th which made me very happy to hear you are all in good health... Here life is still the same, I am still working, it makes the time pass more quickly. I hope you did pay the 1000 F I owe to Mme Ichbia. Incidentally, I used the money here to buy a pair of ankle-high ski boots, they will do me fine for the winter if I am still here. I hope M. Papo is looking into my case as I sent him a message through the social workers and am hoping for an answer. You too, must do whatever

you can, go and see him, as I wrote, and see what can be done...
I hope Bondy, Leon and the children are still well and in good
health...how are Clairette and Marcel? And you, Suzanne, still the
same, busy with needlework? I have been told how you spend every
day sitting in front of the door sewing.

Dear parents, and all the family, I am sending love and affection.

Your son and brother
Michel

A week later, he wrote again, but this time to his sister, Rosa, who was free, this time indicating that his parents were also in the camp, perhaps having arrived just a few days earlier.

Dear Rosette and Paul,

... what a destiny, it is really bad luck having been in camp for
fifteen months...Mama's morale is teffiric (sic), she was so happy
to see me again you can't imagine. Papa is well too, Léon, Bondy
too, the children as well, my bosses all love them already... Take
all you can from the flat, as well as from Bondy's flat, as later
everything will be gone.

Michel

Dear Rosette Paul and the children,

We are all together and our departure has been put off thanks to
Michel. Our morale is better again. I hope yours is too. We are
patiently waiting for events to unfold. I have to ask – and I have no
choice but to burden you with the task – please do all you can and
take as much as you can from our flat, and store the things either
at M. Gouars's or Mme Stambouli's until you can carry them to
yours, before the flat is sealed shut. Have you read the note Michel
sent, and the other small things? Were you, Paul, able to talk with
M. Max about the children? Take the blankets from my place and
mother's, wrap them up into a big parcel together with some soap
and send it in Michel's name with a label... Mama asks me to
tell you to take everything in the way of food. As for the parcel,
it has to be brought to 6 rue de Chaumont, Jaurès Métro station.
Mama has signed a power of attorney so you can collect Edmond's
allowance and send him parcels. At Mama's place, in the shop, you
will find a case full of tins and things to take on the journey...take
everything you can grab, including coal as well as general clothing,

as Bondy said above, that is take them home with you and in the
meantime store them with neighbours. Keep it all, except of course
whatever can be of use to you and wait for news from us... Hurry
up please ... Do not worry, keep calm, we are all quite brave.

Leon

And then on Monday November 10th 1942

Dear Paul and Rosette

... We are leaving in good health, with a strong morale, much in
a hurry. Michel is coming with us. All together...Rosette, go to 9
Rue Richepanse and get a pair of Jamin's ankle boots that was left
for us... the work remains to be paid, and Jean-Pierre can have
them. Do whatever you can to get our two armchairs that were
to be mended on rue Monsieur Le Prince, on the St Michel side,
3/400 to be paid.

Love from Benjamin, Eliane, Bondy, from all of us.

Be calm and brave, you must.

Leon

And then came the 11th of November, of which we know through the
deportation cards the Nazis meticulously filled out, showing that Leon,
Bondy, Benjamin and Rachelle were sent out on convoy No. 45 to
Auschwitz.

   A few days later, and the very last letter in this postmemory narrative is
addressed to Rosa from a person who went to 5 rue le Goff, perhaps just as
Leon had asked. Was there really a way of escaping to the south of France,
as described by Joseph Joffo in his book *A Bag of Marbles*, mentioned in the
introductory chapter?

Melle Denise Ertzlichoff to Paul and Rosette, Paris, Wednesday,
November 16th 1942

... The concierge from 5 rue Le Goff has asked me to say she would
very much like to have news as she liked your sister dearly... As
you have heard, I was at the Broussais hospital where I had been
since October and from which I came out last week. I was being
treated for arthritis of the upper foot and bone decalcification. You
probably heard these details from your sister Bondy as she came
to see me on November 2^d^ with the two little ones on her way to put
flowers on her uncle's grave...So when Melle Froment came to tell

me the dreadful news, how they were all arrested, your poor sister, your brother-in-law, the two little ones, your dear parents, your sister Suzanne, I could not believe in such a terrible misfortune.

Is it possible such things can be done, taking young men away is one thing, we are at war, but women, poor little children and elderly people, it is too horrible, especially in the way the concierge from 5 rue le Goff described it, it is unthinkable and so appalling, your poor sister crashing down on the floorboards with eyes of dread, I am so worried about her health and above all little Benjamin and little Eliane, if they had at least been left with you, or with me, I would have taken care of them and I am sure she would have felt easier knowing them to be safe.

I was told that the friend across from them got a letter in November telling him they were at Drancy, but were going away that very evening to where they did not know.

Maybe you have some news as I heard you were left free though I cannot believe this arrest is about religion, I suppose it is to do with them being Turkish citizens, as I read in the papers about Turkey siding with England and Russia. They should have gone away early in November for I know many who are safe and well in Lyon and Marseille.

I should very much have liked to come to see you and talk in person about all these sad things but I cannot walk and am still in the same state regarding my foot which gives me a lot of pain, and then I worry so much about your sister and the two poor children, they were so sweet.

If you have any news, I beg of you dear Mme Rosette let me know, or if you can come to see me it would make me so happy; hoping you will come – please pass on my regards to your husband...

Denise

That's all that is left. These are the final letters, the ones sent from the one but last stop before the Cohens and the Saüls found their gruesome deaths. Almost the end of the tale. The tale of the Cohen postmemory is drawing to another circle of completion, to be reopened again and again with each remembrance.

While writing this book, there was more than one moment of a flicker of hope, ignited by the question: Was there anyone left alive who could have told the story? Was there anyone else who may have survived, and perhaps did survive?

As the fate of all the Cohens apart from Leon and his family, was not documented, it was impossible or too crazy to imagine that perhaps somebody did survive and managed to escape. Perhaps, Isaac Cohen did manage to use his streetwiseness to flee to the Free Zone and thus survive, like the Joffo story? Or perhaps, one of the two younger brothers who were believed to have joined the Greek partisans? On page 104 of Steven Bauman's book, a Sam (Samuel) Cohen from Salonica is mentioned.[69] Next to it is the date of an interview – April 4th 2003. When I discovered that, in 2016, I immediately wrote to Bauman, asking him for details. He wrote back and said that he has no recollection of that interview but that he will look into his archives, kept in Cincinnati. So far, despite several attempts on my side to encourage him to do so, he has not been able to find that record. The last flicker lost forever? Or was it a wild goose chase to begin with?

Nevertheless, I did my own research and during one crazy February, rang all the Sam Cohens I could find through various phone directories in the USA. Many messages left on answering phones across the continent. I knew that even if it was that Sam Cohen I had hoped it would be, he would be dead, as he was born in 1911. But maybe he had children to whom he had told his story? None surfaced. Nobody answered the call apart from one person who indeed was a relative of a Sam Cohen but bore no relation to a Salonica family. And even he only returned the call from Israel as he was scheduled to arrive there for a wedding and thought that the phone call was to do with that.

That was not the only mention of a Sam (Samuel) Cohen from Salonica I have come across during my research. In the 2020 edition of Isaac Matarasso's memoir, a Samuel Cohen from Salonica is mentioned as one of the few Jews that remained in Salonica after the deportation of the community. He was kept along with eleven other people in a local concentration camp. Isaac Matarasso, who was a local Jewish doctor, who survived by his account thanks to his marriage to a Catholic woman, described in harrowing detail how the "Death Squad" of the Greek police executed those remaining Jews, Samuel Cohen amongst them, on September 9th 1944.[70] Could that have been my Sam Cohen? And if it was, all that I have left is the whereabouts of his death. Which brings the narrative to its last position, the fate of the Cohens in Salonica.

In the beginning of 1943, Adolf Eichmann dispatched two of his agents, SS Hauptsturmführer Alois Brunner and Dieter Wisliceny, to establish "Sonderkommando der Sicherheitspolizei für Judenangelegenheiten in Saloniki- Ägais Kommando," and ordered that Greek Jews should be considered enemies. An order was issued on February 6th 1943 that all Jews were to be marked by a yellow star and they had to concentrate in special ghetto areas.

On March 15th 1943, about 2,400 inmates of the Baron Hirsch ghetto –
a slum Jewish neighborhood next to the railway station – were herded into
forty freight cars overloaded to twice their capacity. Five days later, the
sealed train arrived at Auschwitz. There, after an initial selection, 1,791
men, women, and children were sent immediately to the gas chambers. The
nineteenth (and last) transport left the city on August 10th 1943, with 1,800
exhausted survivors of labour camps. The deportees from Thessaloniki
amounted to nearly 50,000.[71]

Sometime during that period, I have no choice but to see in my mind's eye
a group of my relatives, as they are herded on the carriages. I have been to
that train station more than once. It even has a plaque now commemorating
the transportation. Big deal.

I stood there, gripped with an impossible mix of overwhelming rage and
grief and looked on as in my imagination the Cohens were pushed onto the
trains.

I would like to think that they fought, but I know that they were weakened
after months of near starvation and illness. They could hardly hold themselves together. Still, here they are, on the last procession of death.

First, Henri and Ricetta, his estranged wife who nevertheless could not
but re-join him, and their three children, Shabtai, Morris and Dejo. Henri
gets on last and then offers a hand to his sister, Ines and her husband Moise,
who in turn help their three children, Solomon, also an adult by now, Nelly
and little Rachelle. Next comes Benjamin's widow with her Rachelle. Eli,
right behind her, helps her get on as the shouts of the local Greek policemen
urge them on. I would like to think that Sami and Dino died in battle, with
their brethren partisans. I am there, my dear dead uncles, aunts and cousins
in Salonica and Paris, forever watching you from here, walking alongside
you on that last path, vowing to keep your memory alive.

May your souls find rest.

תהא נשמתכם צרורה בצרור החיים

2020 – An epilogue

Pierre Quillardet, now in his early 90s, still lives in the same building he did when Leon, Bondy, Benjamin and Rachelle Cohen were taken from the house one morning in June 1942. The fact that his testimony is available is uncanny in itself.

In 2008, when the Parentis went to meet with Mireille Florent, Bondy's niece, they also went to visit the apartment on 5 rue le Goff. Without any particular plans, they decided to knock on the door of the flat that Leon and Bondy lived in, sixty-six years earlier. To their surprise, the door was opened and the young Jewish woman who rented the flat showed them in and listened, tearfully, to the reason for their visit. They walked around the flat and asked for the shutter to be opened, so that more light could be let in. It was an intensely emotional time. After about fifteen minutes, another knock was heard on the door, and she let in a middle-aged man, who was obviously in a state of great agitation. This was Pierre Quillardet, who lived across the yard and who just saw the shutters open, after many years that they were shut. He asked the Parentis for the reason for their visit and when he heard they were relatives of the Cohens, he lost his footing and had to be calmed. He then recounted his story, which was documented in a short film made by my father, called *The Green Shutters*. It was an uncanny meeting. Had the Parentis been a day late, they would not have met Pierre, as he was leaving for the summer vacation that day.

Nine years later, in 2017, I visited Paris for a conference of the World Congress of Psychotherapy where I delivered a couple of lectures. I arranged, through Mireille, to meet Pierre Quillardet again in his flat, 5 rue le Goff, and recorded in full our conversation.[72]

PIERRE: *First of all I have a question to you: Why am I so important to you? Why are you so interested in me?*

Q: *Yes, Pierre, before we answer your question, can you introduce yourself, tell us how old are you and say something about yourself?*

PIERRE: *Yes, I was born in 1924, a short time after World War I, in which my father participated. My grandmother married a very famous* architect. *I grew up in a very bourgeois family, with a right-wing political orientation – a conservative family that made sure to give me good values. I was forced to study in a Catholic school where children from families with a high social status also studied. I was raised in a right-wing family, not from the extreme right, but right-wing, so I had no inclination to take care of others.*

Then the war came, suddenly I remember all the anti-Semitic actions I witnessed. My father's sister married a Jewish boy who belonged to a bourgeois Jewish family, where there were many intellectuals. My uncle was a Jew. I was 12 years old in 1936. During this period, during these years, there was very great anti-Semitic propaganda – propaganda that I would describe as a threat. I saw caricatures of Jews, terrible caricatures, and my uncle did not fit in with those caricatures at all. We were friends, he was interested in my studies, he was sporty. The war breaks out and we live under Nazi rule.

Q: *Before we talk about the Nazi occupation, can you tell us your first memories of the Cohen family?*

PIERRE: *I remember them from the time of the war. No, no, I'm wrong. I knew them before the war. I had my own room in my parents' flat, across the yard. One day, it was a beautiful day, I opened the shutters and windows and sat down to do homework, when a boy from the other side – a curly blond boy – shouted at me, "What are you doing?" "Here, you see, I am doing my homework" – that's how our conversations began, from window to window. In winter, we would not talk much. I think we had a difference of seven or eight years. The first time we met and I told him that I was doing homework, he asked me, "What is homework?" So, I asked him, "What, do not you know what homework is?" "No, I don't go yet to school", he said to me. And one day, he said to me, "Well, you know, now I go to school".*[73]

We had quite banal conversations. He was a very cute boy, very funny. I remember that one day he jumped up with joy, and my mother was terrified that he would jump over the window. One day he told me he had a little sister. "What's her name?" I asked him. "Her name is Rachaelle" "And you're happy?" "Yes, I'm happy".

Later, I saw his little sister with him. This was in 1942. That year was the year of my adulthood. In July 1942, we did not live in that flat. After my grandmother's death, my parents decided to live with my grandfather, the architect – in a very large apartment, and from time to time, we would come back here.

One day, I came back and went to the local grocery. I was 18 already. The shopkeeper told me that at night they arrested the Cohen family, who lived on the third floor. We had already heard about such things. We made sure to close the apartment. The guard of the building was anti-Semitic.

We closed the apartment, closed the windows, closed the shutters. These shutters were important to me, and we thought maybe too innocently that when they came back, they would find their apartment – we did not know at all that they had perished in the Holocaust, we thought they were going to work, maybe in difficult conditions but they will be back.

Q: *I'm sorry, Pierre, but to make sure that I understand: You did not live here during this period… You did not see the police coming in the middle of the night and arrest the Cohen family?*

PIERRE: *No, we did not see, we just did not live here, we lived with Grandpa and Grandpa on Avenue de Saxe.[74] We did not see the police, but if we did live here then, when the police came to arrest them, we would not have known because they were arrested at about 2–3 in the morning. The French police received instructions to arrest the Jewish families in the middle of the night, because when in previous cases they came earlier in the evening, around 9–10 PM, the families already knew and could escape. It happened in the middle of the night. But, according to what M. Raye[75] claims, she thinks I would have woken up because when it happened in the middle of the night, there were screams. Yes, the shopkeeper told me they were screaming in the middle of the night. Yes, Mrs. Cohen screamed. They came to arrest people in the middle of the night. Yes, they were arrested and life continued…*

I began my studies. I wanted to become a doctor, a doctor in the navy. I studied in Paris and then went to Rochefort-sur-Mer to prepare for the first year in medicine and to attend medical school in Bordeaux. I also learned to play rugby. I was admitted to medical school, but I had a test and did not pass this test. Because I did not pass this test, I could not continue to study in Bordeaux, so I went back to my parents in Paris. I continued to study medicine in Paris. In my fourth year, I think it was 1946, I met a girl I liked very much. We decided to get married in 1947. My parents still lived with my grandfather. After I decided to get married, I also decided to stop learning. I wanted to work, I wanted to start a family. Luckily, my father-in-law accepted that his son-in-law did not know how to do anything. When he told me, he, who was also a businessman, that I do not know how to do anything, I said: "But I studied medicine", but I eventually admitted that I could not do anything. So, I started working in the chemistry lab, which was affiliated with a pharmaceutical company. I remember that in 1947 I was also a factory worker. I would get up at 7 am and work there, and at the same time, I started working as a representative for the pharmaceutical company, Rosell Labortor.

Q: *And by 1947 you were back here?*

PIERRE: *No, I still lived on Avenue de Saxe with my grandparents. In the apartment at the rue le Goff, a friend of my parents lived there. And in 1948, when I got married, we settled down here and I have lived in Rue le Goff ever since. My wife always said: "I married you because you had an apartment". And so life continued...*

Q: *Well, let's go back to the Cohens.*

PIERRE: *Of course I remembered my conversations with Benjamin. One day, Mr. Saül, Bondy's brother came to me. He came to my parents and told us that they all perished in Auschwitz.*

Q: *When did you learn about it?*

PIERRE: *I think that it was in the 50s.*

Q: *Edmond Saül told you about it?*

PIERRE: *Oh, no, my parents told me. He came to my parents and informed them of the death of the Cohen family. And he asked them to live in their apartment, and they certainly agreed. And when he came to live here, he opened the windows and the shutters. He lived in the apartment for several years. One day, he left the apartment and there were other tenants throughout the years. I stayed in my room across the yard. It was my childhood room and then my son's room, and then it became my office, my study. One day in 1998, I sat down at the table and there was a Jewish woman of Sephardic origin, living in the Cohen' 'apartment, and she never opened her shutters. One day, when I was sitting working at my desk, I looked at the shutters and suddenly I saw Benjamin. And today when I think about it, it's terrible. This boy who was so happy, so nice – how did he suddenly disappear? I felt tremendous pain then, and anger, rage. How such a thing could have happened. And immediately, because I like writing, I began writing a text about Benjamin. I wanted to write, I wanted to tell, I wanted my family to know.*

Then, a few years later, I saw people in the yard talking, so I called the concierge and asked her "Who are these people, what are they doing here?" She told me that they were relatives of people who used to live here... Looking for memories. I told them to come up. That's how I met Mireille and Rony's mother.

Q: *You were present at the plaque ceremony in Benjamin's school.*

PIERRE: *There was Rony's mother and her two brothers. Her brother Benjamin spoke in English at the ceremony. On the same day, Mireille told me that in a school in the 20th arrondissement, signs are being put in memory of the children who perished in the Holocaust, and she told me that she very much wanted us to do so in memory of Benjamin and I agreed. Then, we decided to set up an association with me as the president. Mireille agreed and since then I've been working in memory of the children who perished in the Holocaust. It seems logical to me. I am the president of the associations, the only one there who is not Jewish. And by the way, I have some complaints against my colleagues at these associations...*

As someone wrote: human existence is not a situation we have to suffer, but an honour that we must conquer it. That's what I'm devoting my life to now. It is the Leitmotiv of my life to the end of my days, and I hope it will come soon, I'm sick of it. That's it, more or less how it happened. I do not regret anything.

Q: *This is how it started for you.*

PIERRE: *It was hard work to look for the names of the children, go to all the schools, go to the Holocaust Museum. Yes, we worked hard, we went to all the elementary schools and found 120 names of children. We've even put a sign at the Henri Couture high school. It is a very large and famous school here in Paris. There were seven children and a Holocaust survivor came to testify and explain to the children. The school principals and school teachers did not like the fact that we were putting up a plaque commemorating the children who perished in the Holocaust. It was important to explain, and Maurice Klein, who had survived Auschwitz, did it wisely, gently, without getting into all the awful details. I saw that the children were listening to him. There was also a ceremony at another famous school here in Paris, and it was a very beautiful ceremony, and at the end of the ceremony a history teacher came up and wanted us to do the same in her school, which was a Catholic school in the 5th arr., next to the Paris mosque. She then organized, along with the art teacher, a visit to Auschwitz with her students. But Maurice Klein did not want to come to this school. He would not go to a Catholic school. He kept saying that the Catholics were not so nice to the Jews during the war.*

So, I finally found someone else, also a Holocaust survivor, named Sam Braun – a charming, fascinating man. He fascinated the children and even the school chaplain. They both talked about the existence of the soul, it was very interesting.

Since then, every year, on January 27th, we have been performing a ceremony in the Square René Viviani in Paris. We erected a monument to the children who were too small to go to school, but apparently were not too small to be murdered by the Nazis.

Q: *Why on this date?*

PIERRE: *That's when they liberated the Auschwitz camp.*

Q: *Pierre, when did you understand that the Cohen family would not return at all?*

PIERRE: *When Edmond Saül returned, in 1947. Edmond was a prisoner in 1945, and when he returned, we knew. I went to the Hotel Lutetia to receive all the people who came back.[76] They looked like skeletons. I went to help. I only understood the horror later, because of the shutters, because of Benjamin. I understood when I remembered Benjamin. But immediately after the war, I did not really understand, I did not really understand. I know that my father had a friend, he was a dentist, a charming man, very funny, I really loved going to him to take care of my teeth, and I know that he too perished in the Holocaust. I got the facts then. I did not fully understand what it was about, how difficult it was, how terrible it was. In fact, in 1946, when I was still a medical student in the hospital, we were responsible for anaesthetizing the patients. It was not like today. I remember one day, a woman came in and the doctor told her that she could no longer have children, and she began to cry. I put her to sleep and then saw a number on her hand. During the operation, I started to think that if she came here for hysterectomy, then I realized that she had gone through difficult things in the camp.*

I remember another thing. It was during the period that we call la drôle de guerre[77]. There was some bombing but Germany still had not declared war. This was the year I was preparing my matriculation exams, and my parents decided to send me to Brunoy to a summer camp.[78] This was because I did not study well during the year. When the war broke, my parents left me there.

Q: *Were you in close contact with Benjamin during the 30s?*

PIERRE: *No, I did not see him often. Not in winter, because in winter, I would not open my windows. I rarely met the Cohen family at the entrance to the building.*

Q: *So your only connection to Benjamin was through the window?*

PIERRE: *Yes, sometimes my mother would meet them: 'Shalom – Shalom', and nothing more.*

Q: *Pierre, will there be peace ever? Are you optimistic?*

PIERRE: *I used to be optimistic, not anymore. I am not ashamed to say this: I am a Freemason, I belong to the Grand Orient de France, and I travelled to Israel to establish an order there. I visited the country a little and even planted a tree, I do not remember exactly where, but I remember doing it. We established a group of Freemasons in Israel called 'L'étoile d'Israël' – the 'Star of Israel'. My son, Jean-Michel, was very helpful in establishing the Freemasons in Tel-Aviv, and we did the opening ceremony in Jerusalem.*

I am very philosophical and believe in the philosophy of Camus. He wrote about the absurdity of the world. I am a man of peace. My father was also a man of peace. I want to believe in peace. The point is that today I no longer believe in man. A person has to make a choice and then he has hope. But I have no hope. I feel that I have reached the end of my life, I no longer exist.

I was sitting in Auvergne with two of my sons and granddaughter, and they talked to each other, and I felt I did not belong to this conversation. I do not go out anymore. I think that when my wife passed away 18 years ago, I lost a few things... I tried to live, I played golf... But physically today I'm tired, so maybe that's why my perception of life is quite pessimistic. I'm sick of it.

Pierre is the last known person who can remember the Cohen family. Mireille Florent, Bondy's niece who was in Paris and survived with her family, was only two years old when they were taken to Drancy and Auschwitz. How did her family survive? As is evident in Marianne Leloir's memoir, it was not a subject Mireille's mother was prepared to speak about. In our conversations, we have come to two assumptions: one is the fact that Mireille's father, Paul, was not Jewish and thus spared by the French police on their nightly raids. It is also possible that since the family lived in the 12th arrondissement in Paris, which was less populated by Jews, there were less frequent police raids there. Mireille does remember, or would like to remember, that she had to wear the Yellow Star and was ashamed of it when going to school. She would try to fold her coat lapel over it.

....

What Rita did mostly after the letters stopped arriving, and even after she knew that they were not coming back, was to wait. She waited for her brothers and sister to return, to show a sign of life. She waited for their children to emerge, somehow unscathed, from the catastrophe. Every morning, she reminded her husband, Shmuel, to keep asking around about them. She knew he met many people while working at his market booth at the marketplace. Maybe someone would know, maybe someone had seen them. Maybe a piece of news, a piece of life, would emerge.

And she waited on. She waited for him to return home from the market, usually carrying needed groceries which she welcomed happily. But mostly she waited for him to bring her back something of her family.

She waited, day after day, week after week, month after month, year after year. She died, forty years later, without receiving a single piece of comforting news. No one reappeared, no one had seen them, no one had sent letters. Nothing. A vast horizon of endless anticipation. A desert of lingering and hoping for a figure to appear somewhere in the distance. She strained the organs of her soul to the uttermost but nothing was received. Nothing was noted. The void of the unknown stretched on and on.

Had she lived a mere twenty years more, she would have been there when Mireille Florent was found and with her the discovery of the three boxes of letters, containing many items she would have been overwhelmed to see, to touch, to make sense of. The letters her brother received, the photographs, the documents, the little objects she would have no doubt held close to her bosom as if she were holding him.

Twenty years too late. With her death not only her hopes were dashed, but also ours. She was not there to look through the letters and photographs and give more meaning to their significance. She died and with her died a possible better interpretation of the letters. She could have been the witness who made the letters into a livelier testimony, telling a story that is now forever and truly lost (Figure 40).

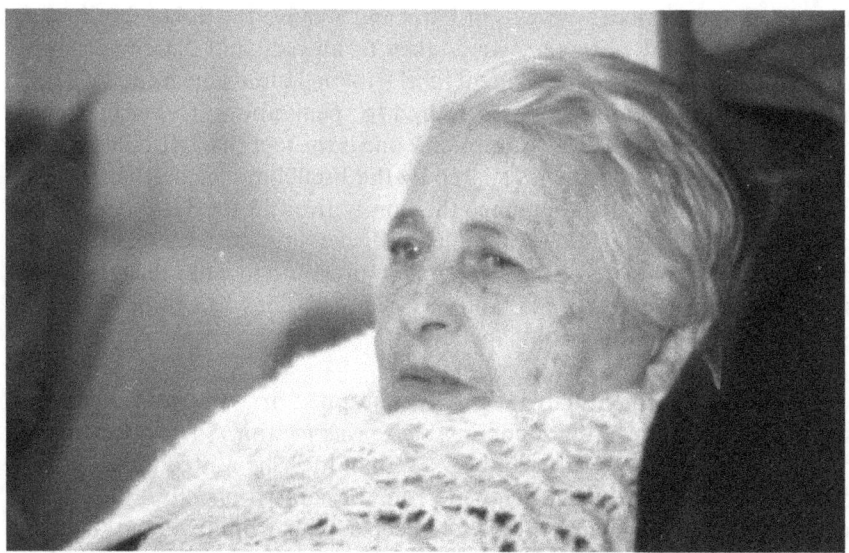

Figure 40: Rita Cohen Parenti.

Notes

1 Steiner, 1997.
2 Mazower, 2005.
3 Naar, 2016.
4 Durrell, 1938.
5 According to Serge Klarsfeld's *Le mémorial de la déportation des juifs de France*, he too was born in Salonica, on February 26th 1897, and like Cohen, was deported to Auschwitz, on June 22nd 1942.
6 Katz, 2015.
7 In his monographs on Jewish Salonica, Devin E. Naar dedicated a whole chapter to the question of how, when, by whom and for what purpose the history of the Jews of Salonica began to be written. He notes, for further reading, see Devin E. Naar, Jewish Salonica: Between the Ottoman Empire and Modern Greece (Stanford: Stanford University Press, 2016), pp. 189–238.
8 Flanner, 1988.
9 Paris, 2013.
10 This is the same letter produced on p. 23.
11 In his monographs on Jewish Salonica, Naar dedicated a whole chapter to the question of how, when, by whom and for what purpose the history of the Jews of Salonica began to be written.
12 The psychic mechanism I am referring to here is called in psychoanalytic terms: *projection identification*. It was explored by the Austrian-born psychoanalyst Melanie Klein (1882–1960), who, like Freud, fled her country once Hitler gained

power and eventually settled in England, where she continued to work after the war. For further reading: Klein, 1975.

13 A listing of telephone subscribers in a specific geographical area, together with their telephone numbers and, sometimes, a street address.

14 Naar, 2016.

15 Bowman, 2006.

16 Joyce, 1957.

17 Is this a reference to a bordel?

18 Bauman, 2009.

19 Kristeva, 1991.

20 Wilson, 1956.

21 Cortázar, 1966.

22 Bakewell, 2016.

23 *Dasein* (in German: *da* –there, and s*ein* – to be) is the term Heidegger introduced to describe his idea of Being as the existential object of philosophical study.

24 Though it is clear that the photo showing Isaac, Leon and Bondy was taken years later, around 1933 or 1934, it is hard not to make a diachronic link between the two references. Perhaps, it took all those years before Isaac was able to make good on a promise he made in 1928.

25 A visiting card carrying her married name, Madame R. Louis Joly, and the invitation to her wedding with Louis Joly on August 15, 1931, are the only indications found so far of the identity of the woman with whom Leon corresponded in those years.

26 Truffaut, 1962, pp. 11–12.

27 Miller, 1935.

28 There are four places bearing the name *Neufchâtel* in Northern and Eastern France. *Neufchâtel-Hardelot*, a farming and tourist town of forests, golf courses and beaches, about 13 km south of Boulogne; *Neufchâtel-sur-Aisne*, in northern France, population in 1931 – 546 people; *Neufchâtel-en-Bray,* in Normandy, northern France and *Neuchâtel-Urtière* in the Bourgogne-Franche-Comté region in eastern France. The name *Neufchâtel* is of course made famous by the *Neufchâtel* cheese, a soft, slightly crumbly, mold-ripened cheese made from cows' milk. In which of the four did Jeanne live?

29 This is the only clue and indication that of the four places with the name *Neufchâtel,* it is perhaps the smallest one, *Neufchâtel-sur-Aisne,* Jeanne lived in as it is nearest to Reims, merely 20 kms away. *Opéra de Reims* was built in 1873. It was rebuilt in 1931, and also served as a cinema, after it was burnt down during World War I, so Jeanne's visit must have been to the new building. It is still open today.

30 An even clearer indication that she was indeed living in *Neufchâtel-sur-Aisne,* a very small village....

31 A selection of small dishes served as appetizers in parts of the Middle East and the Balkans.

32 *Galeries Barbès* was a furniture workshop and shop founded in 1892 on 56 Boulevard Barbès, Paris. Presumably Isaac was doing some business with them.

33 Dowry.

34 Who was she? For the time being, she remains a gaping hole in the fabric of the postmemorial tale. Her story is another *microhistory* left to be unravelled.

35 Yet another relative, another *microhistory,* whose exact connection is unknown. He could have been one of Rachelle's or Shabtai's siblings.

36 On April 25th, Greece decided to abandon the *gold-exchange standard,* like other countries in Europe during the inter-war years and after the 1929 world-wide economic crisis. The Greek economy entered a recession which the Greek financial institutions responded to by anti-inflationary measures, termed *fighting for the Drachma.* For a more detailed report, refer to Chouliarakis' and Lazaretou's 2014 report, issued by the Bank of Greece.

37 The news of Dino's and Sami's conscription is the basis to the assumption, and hope, that they later joined the partisans and were not sent to Auschwitz.

38 A few months later, Rita, Shmuel and the baby girl, would emigrate to Palestine.

39 Shiduch (match-making) is the Hebrew word, also used in Ladino, to describe the traditional process, whereby the parents of young people arrange for a meeting between them, envisaging a good match. It is a social custom still in practice in traditional societies around the world and in different cultures and religions.

40 As both sisters and their mother suffered from pains in their ankles, quite a few letters were exchanged, which were focused on the possibility of Rita sending elastic socks to Salonica. Surprisingly or not, it was easier to buy them in Tel-Aviv than in Salonica. Alas, when the socks did reach their destiny in Salonica, often the postal service damaged them... such mundane preoccupations... which no doubt the sisters were soon to miss.

41 Zmira's given name was first Rachelle but then changed to Martha.

42 Sam Shaki's name would reappear later in letters he wrote from Palestine in the late 1930s, addressed to Bondy. These letters, not included in this book due to its limited scope, indicate that the two knew each other from Salonica. This also explains Benjamin's acquaintance with him and reinforces the assumption that the marriage between Leon and Bondy was based upon earlier family connections formed already in Salonica. Sam Shaki worked in Palestine as a salesman for the Singer Sewing Machine Firm. It seems that he emigrated to the USA from Palestine just before World War II broke out. It is unclear whether he has ever made contact with the Parenti family, as Bondy urged him to do in later years.

43 She must be related to Bondy's family and her visit was towards arranging the wedding reception in Salonica.

44 Between 1931 and 1939, the British authorities issued only 4,000–5,000 immigration certificates each year.

45 This is the only indication that her husband's relatives, the Matarasso family, have also emigrated to Palestine around that time.

46 Bella Parenti was Shmuel's only sister. She emigrated to Palestine a year after Rita and Shmuel with their parents, Esther Evio and Solomon, and settled nearby. She married Isaac Shalom, gave birth to David, Tova and Solomon, who themselves established families in Israel and are living there to this date. Solomon Parenti, Shmuel's father, had three brothers: Simantov, who was childless and emigrated to Palestine and survived, and Elihu and Saul, who stayed in Salonica with their families and perished in the Holocaust. The scope of this book does not allow further study of their lives. They did not leave a single shred of evidence behind them. Not even a single letter was found. The only evidence of their existence is in the Memorial Pages *Daf-Ed,* which Shmuel Parenti registered at the Yad Vashem institute in the 1950s. Of the Evio family, Shmuel's maternal lineage, even less is known.

47 Myasthenia gravis is an autoimmune disease. Today, it is a treatable illness, and most patients recover from it with the right treatment. In the 1930s, however, the mortality rate was 70%.

48 This is probably Dr. Albert Menasche who was also a musician. He was sent to Auschwitz on June 1st 1943, was separated from his family and survived. He wrote a memoir in French where he wrote that it was better to be a musician than a doctor in Auschwitz, as he was made to join the camp's orchestra. See Menasche's 1947 report. In another instance of coincidence, or an expression on the uncanny, the Menasche family figures in Lawrence Durrell's life. His third wife, Claude Vincendon, was Baron Felix de Menasche's granddaughter. Durrell's interest in Jewish life and Israel was not limited to the fact that two of his four wives were Jewish. He wrote the screenplay for Judith, the first international motion picture shot in Israel with American funding, starring Sophia Loren (born 1934) and Peter Finch (1916–1977). The film follows the tale of a young woman, played by Loren, who arrives in Palestine as an illegal immigrant having survived the horrors of the Holocaust in 1944. The location of the production and the filming is set near Kibbutz Shamir. A book version of the script was edited and published by Richard Pine of the Durrell School of Corfu in 2012.

49 She is referring to the attempted *coup d'état* of March 1935, which was motivated by fears of opposition liberal political figures that the government was aiming to give over power to the Monarchists. The coup was unsuccessful, and its leaders were exiled or put to jail.

50 The Maccabiah Games was a sports event held in Mandatory Palestine in commemoration of the 1800th anniversary of the Bar Kokhba revolt, a major rebellion by the Jews of Judaea Province against the Roman Empire. The first Maccabiah took place in 1932 and was very successful. Ines is referring to the second Maccabiah, which apart from being a major sportive event that brought 1,350 Jewish athletes from twenty-eight countries together, also allowed many of them to remain in Palestine, bypassing the strict British emigration restrictions and escaping the worsening conditions for Jews in Europe.

51 Ephetonine is a form of adrenalin preparation.

52 It is a mystery as to whom he may be referring. Could it be one of the Benardout family?

53 Today, that address is a residential street in the 3rd Arr. not far from Lyon Hospital.

54 A Salonica Jewish charity organization that was re-established during the war years and was especially active during the years of occupation. For further details read Kavala's, 2009, Ph.D. thesis.

55 Bondy's brother. Marianne Leloir keeps a framed photograph of him in her study.

56 There have been numerous books dealing with these notions. In my opinion, the earliest one is Wardi, Dina, 1992, *Memorial Candles: Children of the Holocaust*, London: Routledge.

57 Sam Bourla was Rachelle's brother. He married Palumba, and they had two children, Isaac (mentioned in the letter) and Lucy. The family moved to Athens from Salonica before the war. In 1942, they fled to Palestine and thus survived World War II. At the beginning of the 1950s, they emigrated to France. The scope of this book is not enough to do justice to their story. Isaac Bourla married Elza, but they had no children. Lucy Bourla married Albert Molho, and they had two daughters, Nora and Daniele. Nora never married, but Daniele

did and had one daughter, Laurence Molho Kalmanson, who lives in France to this date and has three children with whom I am in contact. I had also met Lucy Molho in 1984 when I visited Paris for the first time. She graciously invited me to stay in her spacious flat on Avenue Salonique, cooked for me lovely dishes that reminded me of my grandmother and, upon parting, gave me a gift of two hardcover books that I keep to this date.

58 Henri Bourla was another of Rachelle's brothers. He too emigrated to Palestine during the early 1930s. He was one of the founders of the Israeli Discount Bank in 1935 and was a very affluent man. Despite that, he turned down requests for help from Rita and Shmuel during the difficult years. No ties were kept with that side of the family. From the letter, it seems that he too spent time in France during the pre-war years. The tone of this letter suggests that they felt judged by him.

59 The change of the name of the city was effected by a Royal decree and was yet another move by the Metaxas government in the process of shedding the Ottoman influence on the city.

60 Shmuel was beginning his work in the Carmel market in Tel-Aviv. First, he was selling merchandise off a tray he carried with him, and then later, he opened a small shop.

61 Prince George's younger brother, Andrew (1882–1944) was married to Princess Alice of Battenberg (1885–1965), great-granddaughter of Queen Victoria (1819–1901) and the mother of Prince Philip (b. 1921), Queen Elizabeth II's husband (b. 1926).

62 Cohen, 2013.

63 Jacques Prévert moved to the Free Zone in the south of France and continued to work with Marcel Carné who stayed in the Vichy zone and continued to work subversively, employing clandestinely several Jewish people and made what would be considered his masterpiece Les Enfants du paradis (Children of Paradise) which was released after the war. Jean Gabin joined de Gaulle's Free French Forces and earned a medal for his participation in the war efforts fighting with the Allied Forces in North Africa.

64 She is pregnant with twins: Rachelle and Benjamin, the two name-bearers of the deceased.

65 It was Benjamin who compiled the first edition of the letters, based upon the first two boxes, with the help of my mother.

66 For a full account read: Chandrinos' and Droumpouki's, 2018, article.

67 These words are the basis for the hope that the two were drafted into the Greek Army and then joined the partisans, thus escaping the fate of the rest of the Jews of Salonica. Somehow, there is comfort to think they died fighting as partisans.

68 For further reading about Drancy, refer to Butler, 1988.

69 Bauman, 2006.

70 Matarasso, 2020. There were dozens of people who went by the name Matarasso that perhaps in the past had some connection. As I checked with Isaac's grandson, François Matarasso, it does not seem that these two Matarassos were linked.

71 Chandrinos and Droumpouki, 2018.

72 The conversation was conducted in French and was translated by my dear friend, Annie Zaouche.

73 The school is located at 12 – 14 rue Victor Cousin, 100 metres from the Cohens' abode. On its wall outside, as well as inside, there's a plaque commemorating the victims of the Holocaust, including Benjamin's name. Rachelle was too young of course.

74 About 3 km south of rue le Goff.

75 The shopkeeper.
76 Today, a five-star hotel in St. Germain.
77 The Phoney war: an eight-month period at the beginning of World War II, during which there was limited military land operation on the Western Front and the French army invaded Germany's Saar district, creating the illusion that the Nazi's progress was stopped.
78 A small Parisian suburb.

Bibliography

Alfandary, Rony, 2019. *Exile and Return: A Psychoanalytical Study of Lawrence Durrell's The Alexandria Quartet*. London: Routledge Publishers.

Alfandary, Rony, 2020. "To be a Refugee: Testimony of a Jewish Bulgarian Family, 1941–1948", in *Refugees from Nazi-Occupied Europe in British Overseas Territories*, Eds. Steinberg Swen and Grenville Anthony. Leiden & Boston: Brill Rodopi, pp. 119–140.

Aymard, Maurice, 2014. "Salonica's Jews in the Mediterranean: Two Historiographical Perspectives (1945–2010)", in *Jewish History*, Vol. 28, No. 3/4, Special issue on Salonica's Jews, pp. 411–429.

Bachelard, Gaston, 1994. *The Poetics of Space*. Boston: Beacon Press.

Bakewell, Sarah, 2016. *At the Existentialist Café: Freedom, Being and Apricot Cocktails*. London: Vintage Books, p. 55.

Bauman, Steven, 2006. *Jewish Resistance in Wartime Greece*. London: Vallentine Mitchell.

Bauman, Steven, 2009. *The Agony of Greek Jews, 1940–1945*. Stanford: Stanford University Press.

Butler, Herbert, 1988. *The Children of Drancy*. Dublin: Lilliput Press.

Chandrinos, Iason and Droumpouki, Anna Maria, 2018. "The German Occupation and the Holocaust in Greece: A Survey", in *The Holocaust in Greece*, Eds. D. Moses and A. Girogos. Cambridge: Cambridge University Press, pp. 15–35.

Chouliarakis, George and Lazaretou, Sophia, 2014. *DÉJÀ VU? The Greek Crisis Experience, the 2010s versus the 1930s. Lessons from History*. Athens: Bank of Greece Publications.

Cohen, Asher, 1996. *The Shoah in France*. Jerusalem: Yad Vashem.

Cohen, David, 2013. "Freud and the British Royal Family", in *The Psychologist*, Vol. 26, No. 6, pp. 462–463.

Cohen, Leonard, 1966. *Beautiful Losers*. St. Albans: Granada Publishing.

Collingwood, Robin George, 1993. *The Idea of History*. Oxford & New York: Oxford University Press.

Cortázar, Julio, 1966. *Hopscotch*, Trans. Greogry Rabassa. New York: Pantheon Books.

Derrida, Jacque, 1960. *Des Tours de Babel*. Paris: Galilee.

Durrell, Lawrence, 1938. *The Black Book*. London: Faber and Faber.

Durrell, Lawrence, 2012. *Judith*. Ed. Richard Pine. Corfu: Durrell School of Corfu.

Felman, Shoshana, 2000. "An Era of Testimony: Claude Lanzmann's Shoah", in *Yale French Studies*, Vol. 97, No. 2, pp. 104–105.

Flanner, Janet, 1988. *Paris was Yesterday*. London: Harcourt Brace Jovanovich.

Fleming, Katherine Elizabeth, 2014, ""Salonica's Jews": A Metropolitan History", in *Jewish History*, Vol. 28, No. 3/4, Special issue on Salonica's Jews, pp. 449–455.

Freud, Sigmund, 1896. "Further Remarks on the Neuro-Psychoses of Defence", in *The Standard Edition of the Complete Psychological Works of Sigmund Freud*, Ed. & trans. J. Strachey, Vol. 3. London: Hogarth Press, pp. 159–188.

Freud, Sigmund, 1899. "Screen Memory", in *The Standard Edition of the Complete Psychological Works of Sigmund Freud*, Ed. & trans. J. Strachey, Vols. 3. London: Hogarth Press, p. 307.

Freud, Sigmund, 1908. "Creative Writing and Day-Dreaming", in *The Standard Edition of the Complete Psychological Works of Sigmund Freud*, Ed. & trans. J. Strachey, Vol. 9. London: Hogarth Press, pp. 141–154.

Freud, Sigmund, 1919. "The Uncanny", in *The Standard Edition of the Complete Psychological Works of Sigmund Freud*, Ed. & trans. J. Strachey, Vol. 17. London: Hogarth Press, pp. 217–252.

Friedländer, Saul, 1978. *When Memory Comes*. New York: Discus books.

Frosh, Stephen, 2019. "Postmemory", in *The American Journal of Psychoanalysis*, Vol. 79, No. 2, pp. 156–173.

Ginio, Eyal, 2002. "Learning the Beautiful Language of Homer:' Judeo-Spanish Speaking Jews and the Greek Language and Culture between the Wars'", in *Jewish History*, Vol. 16, No. 3, pp. 235–262.

Hislop, Victoria, 2012. *The Thread*. London: Headline Publishing Group.

Hoffman, Eva, 1990. *Lost in Translation: A Life in a New Language*. London: Penguin Books.

Ioannou, Yorgos, 1997. *Refugee Capital*, Trans. Fred Reed. Athenes: Kedros.

Joffo, Joseph, 2001. *A Bag of Marbles*, Trans. Sokolinsky Martin. Chicago: The University of Chicago Press.

Joyce, James, 1957. *Letters of James Joyce*, Ed. Stuart Gilbert. New York: The Viking Press, p. 243.

Katz, Ethan, 2015. "Pushing the Boundaries of Mediterranean France", in *The Burdens of Brotherhood: Jews and Muslims from North Africa to France Cambridge*. Cambridge & London: Harvard University Press, pp. 60–110.

Kavala, Maria, 2009. *Thessaloniki during the German Occupation (1941–1944)*. Ph.D. thesis, University of Crete, Rethymno.

Keridis, Dimitris and Kiesling, John Brady (Eds.), 2020. *Thessaloniki: A City in Transition, 1912–2012*. London: Routledge.

Klein, Melanie, 1975. *The Psychoanalysis of Children*, Trans. Alix Strachey. London: The Hogarth Press.

Kokántzis, Níkos, 2003. *Gioconda*. Palermo: L'epos Societa Edtrice.

Kristeva, Julia, 1991. *Strangers to Ourselves*, Trans. L. S. Roudiez. New York: Colombia University Press.

Laplance, Jean and Pontalis, Jean-Bertrand, 1973. *The Language of Psychoanalysis*. London: Karnac Books.

Laurent, Joly, 2018. *L'État contre les juifs: Vichy, les nazis et la persécution antisémite*. Paris: Grasset.

Matarasso, Isaac, 2020. *Talking until Nightfall – Remembering Jewish Salonica 1941–1944*. London: Bloomsbury Continuum.

Mazower, Mark, 2005. *Salonica: City of Ghosts*. New York: Alfred A. Knopf.

Menasche, Albert, 1947. *Birkenau (Auschwitz II), Memoirs of an Eye-Witness: How 50,000 Greek Jews Perished*. Self -Published: New York.

Miller, Henry, 1935. *Tropic of Cancer*. New York: Grove Press, Inc.

Molho, Rena, 1993. "Education in the Jewish Community of Thessaloniki in the Beginning of the 20th Century", in *Balkan Studies*, Vol. 34, No. 2, pp. 259–269.

Montaigne de, Michel, 1588 (2004). *Essays*, Trans. Cotton Charles, Ed. William Carew Hazlitt. USA: Project Gutenberg, p. 53.

Moses, Dirk and Antoniou, Giorgios, (Eds.) 2018. *The Holocaust in Greece*. Cambridge: Cambridge University Press.

Naar, Devin E., 2016. *Jewish Salonica: Between the Ottoman Empire and Modern Greece*. Stanford: Stanford University Press.

Paris, Erato, 2013. *Marseille et Hellénisme (XIXe et début du XXe siècle) [Texte imprimé] : les phanariotes et les néo-phanariotes dans le monde*. Athina: Grafeion dimosieumaton tis akadimias athinon.

Primo, Levi, 1979. *If This Is a Man*, Trans. Stuart Woolf. Harmondsworth: Penguin Books.

Rafael, Shmuel, 2001. "Current Methods and Methodology in Ladino Teaching", in *Shofar*, Vol. 19, No. 4, Special Issue: Sephardic Studies as an Interdisciplinary Field, pp. 85–95.

Reik, Theodore, 1948. *Listening with the Third Ear*. New York: Arena Books.

Saltiel, Leon, 2017. "Voices from the Ghetto of Thessaloniki: Mother–Son Correspondence as a Source of Jewish Everyday Life under Persecution", in *Southeast European and Black Sea Studies*, Vol. 17, No. 2, pp. 203–222.

Saltiel, Leon, 2020. *The Holocaust in Thessaloniki: Reactions to the Anti-Jewish Persecution, 1942–1943*. London & New York: Routledge Books.

Segev, Tom, 2013. *One Palestine, Complete: Jews and Arabs under the British Mandate*, Trans. Haim Watzman. London: Picador.

Steiner, George, 1997. *Errata: An Examined Life*. New Haven and London: Yale University Press.

Truffaut, François, 1962. *Jules and Jim*, Trans. Nicholas Fry. London: Lorrimer.

Wardi, Dina, 1992. *Memorial Candles: Children of the Holocaust*. London: Routledge.

Wiesel, Eli, 1958. *Night*. New York: Hill and Wang.

Wilson, Colin, 1956. *The Outsider*. Boston: Houghton Mifflin Company.

Winnicott, Donald Woods, 1960. "The Theory of Parent-Infant Relationship", in *The Maturational Processes and the Facilitating Environment*. Masud Khan (Ed.), London: Karnac Books, p. 37–55.

Zalc, Claire and Bruttmann, Tal, 2017. *Microhistories of the Holocaust*. New York & Oxford: Berghahn Books.

Zweig, Stefan, (2017) 1938. *Marie Antoinette*, Trans. Eden Paul and Cedar Paul. London: Atrium Press.

Index

Note: *Italic* page numbers refer to *figures* and page numbers followed by "n" refer to notes

How does a person respond to the fact that the formative event of their lives occurred long before they were born? Especially when that event was the Holocaust? In his immensely readable microhistory of the Cohen family from Salonica and Paris, Rony Alfandary skillfully weaves a narrative that grapples with these questions, telling the tales of testimony bearers, human memorial candles of the second and future generations of a family of Holocaust survivors. Listening to voices painfully and suddenly silenced long ago, he uses a treasure-trove of documents to describe and analyze the evolution of "postmemory", showing how it has affected the performative and memorial psyche of survivors' families, continuing on to future generations.

Judy Tydor Baumel-Schwartz, *Director, Finkler Institute of Holocaust Research, Bar-Ilan University, Israel*

Rony Alfandary's evocation of his family's impending fate in 1930s Salonica and Paris is profoundly affective. This collection of letters and photographs is powered by his acute sense of his own postmemory and his professional insight into trauma. It stands beside the work of Eva Hoffman and Sophia Richman as testimony to the perennial sense of Jewish life as (in the words of one surviving relation) "intelligent, loved but unsafe". Alfandary juxtaposes the candid humanity of his family's self-expression with an awareness of difference and "the mystery of Otherness".

Richard Pine, *Durrell Library of Corfu*

In this original and interdisciplinary family history, Rony Alfandary, a clinical social worker, writer and photographer, creates a memorial for the members of his family that perished in the Holocaust. This book takes the reader from Salonica to Paris to Tel-Aviv and back again, on a journey that explores the profound role of postmemory in the lives of those born in the aftermath of the Holocaust. Alfandary is both a storyteller and a therapist, guiding the reader beyond mourning, into a space that allows for creativity and perhaps even joy.

Laura Hobson Faure, *Professor of Modern History and Chair of the History of Modern Jewish Societies at the Université Panthéon-Sorbonne-Paris 1*